Walking Your Way to a Better Life

KIMIKO

VERTICAL.

Translation—Keiko Noguchi
Adam Keys

Published by Vertical, Inc., New York.

Originally published in Japanese as *Pojitibu suicchi!*
by Kodansha, 2006.

Photos courtesy of Keiichi Ohtake; Shufunotomo Co., Ltd.
Illustrations courtesy of Tsugumi Yunagi; Makino Shuppan.

ISBN 978-1-934287-59-0

Manufactured in the United States of America

First Edition

Vertical, Inc.
1185 Avenue of the Americas, 32nd Floor
New York, NY 10036
www.vertical-inc.com

Visit the author's website at
www.posture.co.jp

Table of Contents

Preface

I had a premonition. A vision of a tidal wave of change.

I was 38 years old when I started to teach "posture walking." I have met with great success in just 7 years. I've never been a fashion model and I had very little experience as an instructor. I used to be your average full-time housewife. Now I teach "posture walking" throughout Japan, with bases in Tokyo, Osaka, Kobe, Hiroshima and Okayama. I also hold training seminars for major corporations, and I am involved with educational agencies and intern training programs, and I also collaborate with companies to develop merchandise. I set up an office in New York in 2006.

Considering that I started my first walking class with only 8 students about 7 years ago, the pace of my growth has astonished me. I've been called "Walking Charisma" but I don't like such nicknames. I see mine as more of a self-powered Cinderella story! When it comes to walking, I think that my feelings are stronger than any other person.

The type of walking I teach is not so-called models' "cat-walking" for the runway, nor is it athletic walking with the sole aim of getting into shape. What I aim to teach is the kind of walking that we can all use in our daily lives: walking beautifully and elegantly wherever we go, whether it is to the office, school, or shopping.

There are two points I would like to make:

1. No able bodied person goes through a day without walking at all.

2. Most people seem to be unconscious of the way they walk.

If we start to change the time we spend walking unconsciously into time spent walking elegantly and beautifully, the strain and tension that accumulates during our daily lives slowly evaporates, gradually disappearing all together. This provides a positive effect on both our bodies and our minds.

Walking is a basic function at the root of the mind and the body in humans. This is the main characteristic of the Posture Walking that I teach. I emphasize the word "posture" because what I teach cannot be adequately explained by the word "walking" alone.

Let me go back to the time when it first dawned on me that walking has an effect on the mind. Before I discovered Posture Walking I was a busy full-time housewife with two children. With my mind and time consumed with housework and caring for my children, I felt my sense of self slipping away. I started to catch myself thinking, "I have no time for myself, and nothing to look forward to in the future." This is how I truly felt back then.

Those who lack self-love, and those who carry around certain complexes about themselves, tend to focus too much on outward appearances. One day it struck me that I did not need to obsess over such things. I realized that the one thing that was most important in my life was my body. My body was, and still is, my own fundamental asset.

The mind and body are connected. To harness my mind, I tried new ways of moving my body. By controlling my method of walking, I was able to develop a better understanding of the best way to use my body. I began to feel that every single cell of my body was self-sufficient. This inspired within me the courage to tell myself, "I will keep walking. I will live my life today," and into the future.

I came up with several walking methods to develop the art of self-control.

Although Posture Walking is effective for the superficial goals of slimming down and becoming more elegant, I prefer to focus more on the aspect of raising our awareness and lifting our spirits through the conscious use of our bodies.

In the word "posture" I stress the importance of "mental posture."

I had to pick up my pace in life to get where I am today. Having worked my way up from the very bottom, I know that I have nothing to fear if I find myself having to start from scratch again one day. Some people think that success simply happened to me while I was playing around and enjoying life, and that with luck I ended up the woman I am now. This is not the case.

In my heart of hearts I always knew that I want to live my life as someone who is comfortable in my own skin. There is a flame in me that affirms this conviction, my own personal Olympic flame. It might be small, but it burns brightly inside of me.

No storm, no matter how powerful, can put it out. Like the Olympic torch relay, I want to pass this brightly burning flame on to as many people as I possibly can.

CHAPTER 1

My Story:
The distance from abandoned hope to a new life

Finding Walking

I first discovered walking classes from an advertisement in a local paper. I was 36 years old when I first learned to walk! It seems ridiculous, but it's true. When I saw the flier, I instinctively felt I had to do it.

I wonder why I chose walking classes of all things. When I think back, I'm mystified by it.

I have an aunt who lives in Kyoto. She used to model when she was young. Once when I was a child I went to one of her fashion shows. She made a big impression on me.

"How cool it is to walk in front of an audience," I thought. I still remember how awesome my aunt looked catwalking down the runway. However, at such a young age, anything may have seemed impressive to me.

When I discovered walking, in spite of leading a full life

as a wife, mother and daughter-in-law, I was feeling empty and depressed. I had the feeling that there was something I needed to do, but couldn't quite figure out what it was. So anything that could help clear away the cobwebs of depression would have been okay with me.

Three years prior, I had given birth to my second son, and had gained a lot of weight. My waist stayed at 30 inches after childbirth. My body refused to revert back to the size it was before my second pregnancy figure. Though I was vaguely aware that my body had grown dumpy, one day one of my friends showed me a picture that we posed for together. I was astonished to see the reality of just how bad it had gotten.

I felt like I'd been slapped.

"Is this *me* in the picture?" I was so shocked, I felt as though I wanted to take off my body and throw it away like an old, worn-out dress.

After a while though, I was busy again taking care of my children, and I couldn't find the time to go to a gym. I tried dieting with little success. I waited until my second son was three years old.

"Since walking seems so easy, it's probably easy to stay on course." With this thought in mind, I started taking walking classes. The teacher of these classes used to be a model that worked with a top modeling agency. She was one year older than me. She had even features, a good figure, and was about 5'9". She was very cool.

"She's so pretty! How can we be so different even though we're both human beings?" I always looked at her with envy.

It was a two-hour lesson once every two weeks. At the beginning I practically worshipped the teacher, feeling happy to be able to breathe the same air as her.

Walking itself also enchanted me. I found myself filled with a feeling of refreshment that is almost indescribable. I continued to take lessons even though I only had a small amount of free time.

"It feels so good just to walk with good posture!"

At first, I was more surprised by the change in my feelings than the changes in my body. Waking helped me become more and more positive. I think the pleasure of walking I was feeling in those days was a realization that I could take time for myself; and that was very enjoyable.

If I had just ten minutes a day to walk, it was "me" time. As I was focused on raising my children and trying to be a good mother, wife and daughter-in-law, I didn't have a whole lot of time just for myself. But when I could, I walked. It felt as though I was on a date with myself! It was an enormous pleasure among the day-to-day hustle and bustle of my life.

After that I worked to redress my posture and walk

beautifully every day. When I shopped, or when I hung the laundry, I focused on my posture. After I sent my children to school and sat down to eat, I held my torso upright, imagining that I was in a fancy restaurant.

I realized one day that I was developing my own ideas about walking methods.

Time to pounce

I think I'm greedy by nature.

After each lesson term was over, I signed up for whatever class that same teacher was doing next. I took the same courses again and again without ever getting tired.

Since I liked my teacher, it was almost like I was her groupie. I kept taking her classes for two years.

Finally, I started to feel dissatisfied with learning the same walking lesson again and again. At that point, my teacher said, "You can walk perfectly fine now, so don't you think you can give up these lessons? It's not like you're ever going to be a model or anything."

I was very shocked by the way she pushed me away.

But looking back, her attitude had always been like that. If was as if she thought, "I am a model. You are mere house-wives. Don't forget that." Although that was true, of course, I didn't think that she should look down on her students or think she was somehow better than us. However, hearing her words helped me to wake up from the spell I was under.

I suddenly realized that I loved walking itself more than she did. I thought, "I get far more pleasure from walking than she does!"

By that time, a dramatic improvement in my figure had already taken place. My waist had become three inches slimmer, and I had become thinner and more toned overall. My height had increased a full inch. When I began, I hadn't expected such major changes.

"You look like you've had full-body plastic surgery," people said. I thought so, too.

I used to have a typical middle-aged figure before I started walking lessons. Why had my body changed so much just by changing how I walk? Just by being aware of my posture in my daily life, without ever using a surgical knife or putting a foreign object in my body, my looks had totally changed. This led me to explore the possibilities of walking, and it enchanted me more and more.

Since my teacher used to be a professional model, she had probably never had the experience of struggling to lose weight, or suffering from having no time for herself or having a terrible complex about her body. I think she missed out on the experience of being rescued by walking.

I was the total opposite. I had an inferiority complex about my body, and I thought, "I'm so big and my life's so small." I couldn't make use of the body that I was born with. I couldn't find clothes that suited my tall figure. I disliked my body.

But I found so much happiness through walking. "If I were a teacher, I could tell my students about my experience. It's only a dream, but I want to be able to help others." I felt a new conviction.

"I love walking more than my teacher, and I am more grateful for the benefits of walking than she'll ever be." I was proud to think that I had more regard for walking than she did.

Then, it happened. I became a teacher.

My best friend since high school also practiced classical ballet as a hobby asked me to teach.

Having witnessed the change in me, she felt that my progress was amazing. She had a particular understanding of how difficult it was to develop beautiful back muscles, having practiced ballet for many years herself. She knew me from when I was single, and she saw how my body had drastically changed from the weight gain after I'd given birth to my sons. She's known me through all my ups and downs.

"Kimiko, walking has changed you! You're so cheerful, healthy and strong now!" she said. "Why don't you teach the walking method you've learned at the child care center where I work as a secretary?"

I hesitated at first. "Me?" I asked. But then, I decided to give it my all.

It became a major turning point in my life.

Memoirs of an average housewife

I was born and raised in Okayama prefecture in western Japan and graduated from an all-girls high school. I came to Tokyo when I was transferred to the Tokyo office of the organic cosmetics company that I was working for at the time.

I was 27 years old when I got married. The opportunity to get married came about when a client introduced me to the man that would be my future husband. Since the company was selling cosmetics, most of my clients and co-workers were women. Knowing my life was devoid of much male company, the client worried about my prospects for marriage.

"I'll introduce you to a good man who is the son of the owner of a company where I used to work. Would you like to meet him?" Already 26, there was little hope for me finding a partner if I was surrounded by women all day at work. "You'd better marry while you're still young and beautiful!" the client said.

Though I did dream of getting married—more so than

most women my age—it was just six months after I had moved to Tokyo, and I was about to be given more responsibilities at work. I was hesitant. In the end I decided to meet him, figuring I shouldn't take it too seriously. "It might be nice to have a boyfriend," I thought.

My future husband was being groomed to inherit a certain company in Tokyo. He was very kind, and he created a warm ambience wherever he went. After our initial meeting, we started dating.

We went to a very famous sushi restaurant on our first date. It was an expensive restaurant often frequented by celebrities. Pretty impressive, right? My family rarely ate out back in Okayama, so it seemed very luxurious to spend money that way.

"I could get used to a life like this," I thought to myself happily. People around me often said, "You should marry a rich guy and ride the gravy train." I realized it might not be such a bad idea.

I was also keen to relieve my parents' worries. If I married him, I thought, he would take good care of our family and give a sense of stability to my life.

Our original meeting was premised on seeing whether marriage was a possibility, so the decision for us to date was already a lead-up to the big day.

When I met him, he was 32 years old, and people were anxious for him to hurry up and get married. When he invited me to his home, his parents welcomed me very warmly. We decided to get married soon after. But it wasn't until after the wedding that I realized, "Tokyo is a big, modern city, but I've married into a very old-fashioned family."

We had a grand wedding reception. When we returned from our honeymoon, he brought me around to meet all of his relatives. Because many of the neighbors had lived in the area for a long time, they were a very tight-knit group. When I went shopping, I always ran into someone who knew my husband. I always had to stop and exchange pleasantries with them.

One day I had a cold, so I went out to the store without bothering to put on any makeup. Some days later, my mother-in-law told me that a neighbor gossiped to her that I was seen makeup-less in public. I was shocked that they would care about such a thing.

But I had no complaints about my home life. My husband was faithful and a hard worker, and my in-laws were very good people. I thought that it was selfish of me to feel dissatisfied.

"Fit in with this family." "Don't embarrass them." "Try to be the beloved new daughter of this house." I always thought such things.

I helped with the office work in the family company from morning until evening while I was pregnant with my first son, right up until the month I was due. I performed these duties because it was appropriate and proper for the bride of the eldest son in the family. Even after giving birth to my first-born, I helped in the office once he was in kindergarten.

When my first son was born, my in-laws' joy was considerable.

Ever since he was born, they referred to him as "the third generation." All the neighbors were very pleased about this too. For my in-laws, he's the heir-to-be of the company they had founded, so he was—and still is—the apple of their eye, and is seen as their most significant grandson.

For him, the memory of being loved by his grandparents seems to be very strong. His grandparents would take him to a local candy store, or give him pocket money, telling him to keep it a secret from Mommy. I had mixed feelings about such things, but I wanted to respect the feelings of his grandfather and grandmother.

Recovering from resignation

I laugh when I think about it now, but in those days I was very envious when I saw friends who dyed their hair. I thought they were lucky to be able to do such a thing.

"What would my mother-in-law say if I dyed my hair?" I thought to myself.

My mother-in-law wasn't a person who made unreasonable or strict remarks, but because she was born before the war, she was a little conservative in that she wanted me to lead a quiet and discreet lifestyle. I wore the clothes my mother-in-law bought for me, or hand-me-down sweaters from her. Because of this I looked old and frumpy. I thought that it was my fate to live in a manner that complied with my mother-in-law's will. I was glad to be thought of as a good bride, so I desperately tried to mold myself to her ideal.

My mother-in-law was a good cook. When I learned that my husband liked his mother's *nukazuke*-style pickles, I worked hard to perfect the technique. I disliked the sweet Tokyo-style omelet that my mother-in-law made, but as it was "the taste of home" for my husband, I learned how to make it.

"This makes my husband happy." "This makes my father-in-law happy." While I was thinking that these things constituted my happiness as well, there were also vague, ill feelings forming in my heart.

It was around this time that I found about walking lessons on a flier inserted in the newspaper.

I almost gave it up as soon as I saw it. "There's no way

they'd let me leave my kids at home and go out just to learn a new hobby," I thought. However, I found it difficult to totally extinguish my desire to try something new.

I made up my mind to leave the door to my yearning slightly ajar.

Awakening to Teaching

"Keep your head up and back!" "Swing your arms further behind you!"

Since I discovered Posture Walking, my buried feelings came to light. My dreams and my ability to think about the future became clearer and stronger within me.

Walking is the only thing I can think of that caused these changes. Until then, I always tried to meld into my environment. I was convinced that it was selfish to express myself honestly. However, I was awakened to the joy of finding expression through walking. I learned the joy of finding my own walking method and of proper body use.

My walking lessons that had begun with a helpful push from my friend were extremely well received. I taught about eight mothers in a tatami-style room in the community center next to where some toddlers played or napped.

I was in high spirits: "I'm a teacher!" I taught my lessons while dressed in a showy-yet-neat outfit. Everybody always complimented my style. That made me happy.

Some of them said, "We'd love to have you teach a longer course." So I rented a studio in Fukuo and taught a six-part course. It was my first class. This was in 1999.

I'll never forget the studio on the second floor above an old bar. It cost me about 7000 yen (around $70) per session. The lesson fee was 1500 yen in those days, so I only pocketed about 3000 yen after I paid the studio charges and sundry expenses, even if ten students came.

I remembered that I very carefully smoothed out the first 3000 yen I had earned and put it away in one of my drawers.

Even in those early days, I was mysteriously confident. I knew that our bodies have infinite possibilities, and that the future is something we create for ourselves. Walking lit me up, physically, mentally and emotionally. My students slowly began to find joy in themselves as well.

"You're lovely, and I'd like to see you again. You're the ideal woman for many of my friends who are also mothers." I often received such compliments.

"I'm being useful to other people," I thought. Not just as a mother or a wife, but as an individual. I felt like I was accepted as myself for the first time. Making money was not my first priority.

My life was parched. I went to the studio and I found an oasis. I was really happy.

"It's ten years too soon for you to teach!"

My first walking teacher, as I mentioned before, was a model. I was enthralled to her. But there came a time when the spell was completely broken.

When my friend asked me to teach at the community center, I asked the teacher if it was okay for me to teach.

"The nerve you have got!" she laughed at me with her nose turned up. "Let me tell you something. It's impossible for a person like you, a housewife, to make a living in this business. Just because you can walk a little better than others doesn't mean you're ready to teach anyone. It's not that easy."

I was stung. But then I thought determinedly, "I *will* make a living by teaching walking!" From that point on, I started to keep my distance from her.

Around that time there was another woman who tried to knock me down. One day, I took a class with a certain teacher who was leading a course in face yoga. I had taken such a class before and wanted to learn more.

The teacher was a middle-aged woman. From the way she dressed, I could tell that she worked in the fashion industry. She had a stout build, but she had a dignified presence that made her seem fascinating.

Because I had just started teaching my own walking classes, I was enthusiastic about getting the word out. I held out my business card and the brochure I had made for my classes and introduced myself. "I actually learned walking from Ms. So-and-So."

"Oh, I know her. She occasionally models for me." The subtext was, "I'm far better than she is."

The next day, I got a call from her.

"It's presumptuous of you to teach others when you have only been taking classes for just 2 years. Before that you were just a housewife, weren't you?"

There was a reason why the teacher was angry with me. The profile that I had handed her said, "I teach walking, proper movement and face yoga."

I also wrote that I learned face yoga from the competition. Although I didn't mean to offend her, I can understand how she may have seen that as an affront.

"You don't seem to understand that during face yoga, students contort their faces in various ways. If someone were to develop wrinkles they could try to sue you. And by the way, I don't think you walk very well at all. You need way more classes. It's ten years too soon for you to teach!"

Her words depressed me greatly. With the receiver still

in hand I slumped down onto the floor, my mood darkened.

"Because everyone knows everybody in this small industry, I'm sure you'll be beaten down if you try to take it on now. I'm telling you this for your own sake, you know. You can start teaching after you receive more tutoring from me."

However, there were students who were truly pleased with my lessons. One of my friends said, "There are people like her everywhere. She's just getting territorial, and she probably enjoys tormenting people younger than she is."

Hearing such things was very encouraging. But through this experience, I realized that I was trying to go in the wrong direction.

In those days, I was teaching walking to aspiring models and actors. I felt like I had to stretch myself and act like I was on par with members of the entertainment industry. When I taught lessons to young models, I was often asked, "Did you use to be a model?" There were some friends who said, "Why don't you just say that you're a former model?" I myself had also thought that it somehow looked bad to say, "I was just a housewife." Plus, I thought setting the record straight was a hassle. I thought that it was okay to lie and tell them, "I was a model."

With all the compliments I received, I was probably overly confident. However, I suddenly felt that since I knew nothing of the world of models and actors, I shouldn't try to act like I did. Many people long to be a part of showbiz, but it's no place for me.

What I should aim for, I realized, was to let ordinary people like me discover the splendor of proper walking.

At that point I developed a firm resolve. Walking that can be done anytime, anywhere—the idea of anyone, from children to the elderly, being able to rediscover the pleasures of walking and to incorporate my methods into their daily lives was the concept that suddenly and strongly took root in my heart.

Therefore, I intend to thank my first walking teacher and the face yoga teacher if I run into them somewhere sometime. Their words became the major guideposts for my present direction in life.

Divorce

After I discovered Posture Walking, I became incredibly positive. There was a time, however, when I felt as though I was going to worry myself to death.

Divorce.

Originally the idea was that my husband and I would eventually take over the family business. It irked my husband and my in-laws that I began working independently as a walking instructor. Even so, my passion for teaching did not diminish. Deep down, though, I was conflicted.

"Will it be good for my husband and his family for us to stay married?"

It was impossible for me to teach walking just in the short breaks I could take while devoting most of my time to the daily challenge of running the family business. I thought that if I was going to teach, I needed to focus entirely on teaching and give it my all.

But I held back, as I had to consider the welfare of my children.

After battling myself daily for 2 years, I had a heart-to-heart discussion with my husband. I talked about getting a divorce. At that time there was no guarantee that I could make a living on my own just by teaching walking. But after quite a bit of introspection, I couldn't deny the feeling that this was what I needed to do.

I put an end to my married life of 13 years, which started when I was 27 and ended when I was 40.

A woman is strong once she commits to her choices.

"I will work hard. I will make money," I told myself. I persevered with all my heart. Whenever people do their absolute best, life's doors open one after another.

Even now, I have only feelings of appreciation towards my

ex-husband and my former in-laws. At the end of the divorce process, we shook hands and parted amicably. Nowadays, we occasionally dine together. He's still the father of my two children, after all. We still cooperate on raising our children.

Also, if I hadn't had the experience of being a housewife, I may never have discovered Posture Walking.

Days spent running up the stairs

One day soon after I became newly independent, no students showed up for one of my lessons. I was all alone in the ballet studio that I rented out for the class. I was disappointed for a moment, but I tried to cheer myself up focusing on my figure as I saw it reflected in the giant mirror of the studio.

I was mysteriously refreshed and the fog in my head cleared. I danced and moved my body while looking in the mirror, and gradually various ideas about walking and movement bubbled up inside my head.

There were hints of a new walking method that lay dormant in my own body. I realized this, and I was suddenly obsessed with finding out what it was. I communicate inwardly with my body, and this reveals the pathway to me.

It was spring in 2002 when I learned the English word "posture."

I was teaching a walking class to students at Hosei University. A female student who was taking lessons talked about them to her American boyfriend. When he heard that she was talking walking classes, he said he found it absurd that Japanese people would spend money to learn how to do something as basic as walking. So she straightened up her back and walked with her head held high to show him what she had learned.

He said, "Oh, that's *posture!*"

When I heard this, it was as if an electric current had run through my body. I sensed, "That's it!" It was the word that I needed, since I wasn't able to express the concept fully by using the term "walking" alone.

There's a key characteristic of the type of walking that I teach. And it was that moment that I realized what it was: mental posture.

In 1999, I first started teaching classes in Fukuo. In 2001, an article ran in *Tokyo Shimbun* (Tokyo News) and the number of students taking my lessons suddenly shot up.

In 2002, I registered a trademark for the names "posture walk" and "posture stylist" (currently pending in the U.S.A.). In 2003, my first book was published.

In 2005, I taught my first class overseas in New York. In 2006, I established an office there.

I still occasionally find myself thinking back to the days when I was an average full-time housewife. I particularly remember a dream that I had one night when I was 32. In the dream, I was 37 years old, not 32. "I'm 37...but I haven't done anything of importance!" I dreamed. I was terribly sad. After I woke up, at first I was relieved to still be 32, but then I felt very strongly that I had to start doing something. "I can't stay this way forever!" I thought.

What was that dream hinting at? Well, just before I turned 37, I discovered Posture Walking.

"What will change just by changing how I walk?" "What's the difference if I fix my posture a bit?"

I still get such questions all the time. However, learning proper walking changed my life. It made the core of my life thick, sturdy and very, very strong.

CHAPTER 2

Methods for the Mind

Method 1: Turning on the Positivity Switch

I have been able to change my life by having my "positivity switch" permanently on.

It was through Posture Walking that I was able to naturally acquire the ability to turn on the switch. This is the only reason for the change.

When I have my picture taken with my students, I shout, "I'm pretty!" instead of "Cheese!"

In the morning before I leave the house, I look in the mirror and compliment myself. "You look perfect!" "You look so cool!" When I walk, I say to myself, "I feel great!" or "I am in great shape today!" and pace my walking to the rhythm of the positive words in my head.

At the beauty salon, when my stylist asks me, "How would you like your hair cut today?" I reply, "Make me the most beautiful person in the world." Seems funny, doesn't it?

Though I'm half-joking, my stylist, who is familiar with my method, sincerely replies, "Got it!" and cuts my hair eagerly. This makes me feel as though I am gradually becoming the most beautiful woman in the world, with each snip of the scissors!

Once the positivity switch is on, positive energy will start circulating and gaining momentum as if it's a ball rolling down a hill. Does that sound strange? Give it a try. I promise there's nothing to lose, and you won't regret it.

The heart has feelings, but so does the body. If you treat your body with care, it will respond with joy.

"I feel great!" "I am perfect!"

If you keep telling your body these things, your body will react positively to the words, just as negative phrases like "I am worthless" will bring negative feelings into your body. Your body will naturally react to your words, whether positive or negative. The connection between words (even if they're only in your head!) and the body is very interesting.

Saying "I *want* to be beautiful" is not enough. Wishing to be a certain way only tells your body that you're dissatisfied with yourself as you currently are. Affirming that "I am beautiful" in the present tense turns on the positivity switch. Make saying such things to yourself a habit.

The realization that you are totally alive will surface

strongly once you begin to think and act in your own rhythm. What is this rhythm? It's how you walk. Every day we walk, mostly unconsciously. The way we walk is an expression of our personal inner rhythm.

So changing your walk to a more beautiful method means changing the length of each stride, the position of your eyes, and the way each muscle is used, all of which change the rhythm of movement of the body, making you more beautiful. Changing the rhythm will also change your pattern of thinking.

If you keep doing this every day, it will change your life. This is because the mind and the body are one.

By discovering the concept of Posture Walking, almost without noticing, I experienced this step. Imperceptibly, I kept turning on the switch in the "spine" of my mind. Then, wonderful things happened! My life unfolded before me. I have the confidence to recommend this to anyone because of my very positive experience.

Method 2: Discovering the beauty within you

I started walking consciously when I was 36 years old. At that time I thought, "I have no future." While raising my children, I felt my body growing ugly. With all the housework, my hands were worn down. I did not have time to indulge myself. I felt my womanliness was starting to wilt and die off. I think that I truly hated myself at that time. However, after starting to walk effectively, light began pouring into my life.

I adapted something called "image training" for use in my lessons.

I based the lesson on my own experiences. It sounds a little difficult at first but it's actually very easy. It's a game where you list 100 aspects of your beauty on a sheet of paper. The aim is to identify and label your beauty in a specific manner, and then write each aspect down.

"My eyes are beautiful." "My voice is beautiful." "My collarbone is beautiful." "My skin is beautiful," etc. The aim in doing this is to discover your beauty and turn on the positivity switch.

In the case of a course spread over six lessons, I usually ask my students to do this as an assignment during the third lesson, and the students bring in their completed lists for the fourth lesson.

At first, every student reacts the same: "Oh, no!"

They complain, saying, "This is pointless." They feel that they're being forced to do something crazy, with some saying, "I can't do such an embarrassing thing!" or "I'm so busy. I can't afford the time for that."

They put up quite a lot of resistance. Especially the

men—the majority of them are like that. However, the right approach is to say, "It sounds ridiculous but I'll give it a try!" Though only the people who have tried this exercise can truly understand, it turns out to be very pleasant work.

People say, "At the beginning, I wrote this in secret so that nobody would see it." But then they say, "I was eager to finish it!" or "I slowly became obsessed with it!"

I use this exercise during seminars for major corporations. Middle-aged men come around to admit, "I'm starting to feel like I'm actually attractive," and they really get into the game. When I ask, "Doesn't it make you happy?" they answer, "You know, I actually do feel happy!"

This is an example that shows how most of the time we fail to listen to our body's feelings. Our body is very sensitive and wants much more attention than we typically give it.

I think many people these days lack this kind of balance between the body and the mind.

Method 3: To people who do not like themselves

When I talk about image training, I'm reminded of a student I once had.

She was a married woman in her 50's. I asked her to do the 100 beauty aspects exercise. Though she was tall and lovely with cropped hair, she said, "I really cannot write anything positive. I am stuck for words."

However, I encouraged her. "Please try your best to write. If you don't do it, you'll have to come up with 200 instead of just 100."

So finally, after mustering her courage, she made the list. Then she told me the reason that it was so difficult for her at first.

Since she was little, her parents always said to her, "Your sister is pretty, but you are not, so we will let you put on pretty clothes to make up for it." She had lived her whole life up until taking my class assuming that it was wrong for her to think of herself as beautiful. "I don't belong in the world of beauty," she thought.

However, because of the homework I set, she started to think about herself while she reluctantly began her list. While she was writing, tears started to run down her face as she realized that she was allowed to think of herself as someone who is beautiful. She realized this fact for the very first time. She told me that she realized how she had been bound by the words and value system imposed by her parents. As she told me all this, her face turned bright red.

On hearing her tell me these things, I cried. We both cried, holding each other's hands. The words spoken by parents to their children are extremely powerful and influential.

Long ago, I assumed that I had to give up my beauty in order to be a good housewife. However, the world changed for me completely after I was able to find the true beauty within myself. Everything became brighter and the scenery around me burst into color.

People often think or tell themselves things that aren't good for their bodies. I want everyone to stop saying abusive things to their bodies.

At the same time, I think people today have a wall up to protect themselves against complicated words. Yet we have a weakness against simple complimentary words that strike right through the walls we put up around ourselves.

People who try to keep up a tough façade are especially vulnerable to the effect that very simple words have on their hidden, tender hearts. Those who always have the last word in complicated arguments are easily flattered when they are told that they are "Wonderful!" or "Cool!"

"Beautiful!" "Fun!" "Nice!" "Happy!" People melt like butter when they are complimented with these kinds of words. In general, people don't use positive words in regards to themselves. Instead they bind their body with negative feelings and complicated words.

Even so, deep down, I think everybody likes at least some aspect of his or her body. You want to like your body but can't. So I think that if you direct positive thoughts and words towards your body, things will change for the better.

You need to turn on the positivity switch in your mind.

Turning on this switch gave me a sense of readiness. I developed a physical constitution that doesn't have room for regrets. I don't know exactly why, but the full awareness and joy of being alive began to flood through me. My mind switched to the positive.

To achieve this state you must change your habitual thought patterns.

Method 4:
The motions that bring about a turning point

I'll never forget what started me on the road towards fame in Japan. It was an article that ran in the evening edition of the *Tokyo Shimbun* on September 25, 2001. The article had a large spread of photos showing walking lessons at my school in Meguro, Tokyo, which I operated in those days.

The response to the article was impressive. Up until then, I had only gained students through word of mouth. After the article appeared, 100 new students signed up immediately, and from then on the numbers continued to swell.

This turning point in my life came about through a special encounter.

At a concert I attended one night a middle-aged woman who was sitting next to me suddenly turned and looked me up and down.

"Can I help you?" I asked.

"What do you do? You must be doing something special. Am I right?" she asked.

I gave her my card and told her that I taught walking. She said, "In that case, I'll get my friends together for a group lesson, if you wouldn't mind teaching us."

The woman happened to be the president of a cosmetics company.

Inspired by the woman's interest in me, I rented a classroom in Meguro for her group's lesson. Many of the students were of a certain age, and one of the students was acquainted with a journalist for the *Tokyo Shimbun*.

She wrote that the lesson was different from her pre-conceived notion of what a walking class was. She imagined that the lessons were going to be about catwalking or athletic power-walking. However, it turned out to be something that "anyone can take up in their daily lives regardless of age." This statement made the response to the article particularly impressive.

I often notice that there are many of these kinds of random encounters that lead to turning points in life. A woman working at a publishing house, who happened to take a walking lesson, led me to the opportunity to release my first book, *Beautiful Walking Posture.*

Another such person was Tome Kamiooka, who drew the illustrations for my first two books, and introduced my walking lessons in her own books. These mentions were like ads for my lessons.

This circle of people all mysteriously connected and produced a positive effect. However, I think such occurrences happen to anybody involved in any line of work. For instance, when you consider asking someone to do a task for you at work, what first comes to mind is, "I'd like *so-and-so* to do that for me."

When it comes to co-workers, I'm sure that everyone wants to work with people who are pleasant. If you had a choice, would you want to work with someone whose back is hunched over, who's hiding their face behind their hair?

When I hold training seminars for companies, I often talk about nonverbal communication. Everybody communicates with others before they even open their mouth.

This is because our bodies give off signals. Your body is in fact far more communicative than you probably realize. If you look at it from such a perspective, someone whose body language is attractive is more likely to do well in business.

The act of brushing up your body language starts with awareness of your spine.

Your spine is at the center of your body and is therefore the center of your movement as well. If your spine is held up correctly, your movement is more beautiful, and if you keep an attractive posture, your body language naturally appears more polished and refined.

Walk beautifully. Acquire a beautiful posture. Create an attractive body language. Then the signals given off by your body will automatically become more beautiful.

I think there are people that have more luck than others, but if you really think about it, in most cases such people have called fortune towards them with their own will. Except in cases like winning the lottery by pure chance, "fortune" is something you attract to yourself.

So walk with your face raised, chest open, and heels landing firmly on the ground. Live—and walk—with confidence. Positive feelings will begin to well up in you.

Method 5:
The power of the imagination can change your life

Since that fateful article in the *Tokyo Shimbun*, I have received a fair amount of media exposure. And I never went looking for it! Prior to the article, I only occasionally put a small ad in a local news magazine, which cost about 4000 yen for just two lines of text.

However, I had had a premonition that things would get to this level from a while back. Because I have confidence instilled in me from my Posture Walking, I know that I have the power to create a bright future for myself.

I also began to notice the importance of the imagination. For example, when I was given the offer to write my first book, the first thing I did was to look for a fountain pen. I fantasized about how cool it would be to sign my name with a flourish of a nice fountain pen once my book was published.

I decided that I needed one, even if it was expensive. After asking the store clerk questions for nearly three hours, I finally decided on a very nice fountain pen. I felt from the bottom of my heart that I had to get that particular pen. However, I didn't buy the pen at that time. (The clerk nearly fainted from disappointment!)

"My book will be published this fall. I'll come back and buy the pen then," I announced.

So I worked diligently on my manuscript, with the image of the perfect fountain pen in my mind like a carrot before a horse.

It's not healthy to depend too much on physical possessions, but there are times when they can assist you. The important thing is how to make proper use of them.

When I go shopping, I always picture precisely what I want to buy in my mind before heading out. Then if I find a close match to what I envisioned in a store or display window I buy it right away. Walking around not knowing what I really want just makes me tired.

I bought a handbag in this way as well. I knew that I wanted a shoulder bag that could fit A4-size documents. One day, I saw such a bag in a store window. I thought, "That's it!" I bought it then and there.

When you're shopping for something new, you really shouldn't look at the price tag first. When you finally look, if it's too expensive for you to buy right then and there, think something like, "I will come back and buy this one day when I have become a version of myself that can afford this." Never compromise.

In my desk drawers at home I have several jewelry catalogues. Even though I don't possess the actual jewelry, the effect of having the catalogues is the same as having the real thing. The images alone make me feel rich.

Thinking, "I can't afford it!" is different from thinking, "I'll be able to buy it someday."

It's important to steer the direction of your words and thoughts towards the positive, whatever the circumstances.

Consciously choosing the way we react to an incident will change how we feel about it.

Our feelings create our mood and ambience. So if you visualize your self and possessions as being very first-class, you will give off a high-end vibe.

I use the same method in my work as well. "I'm sure such-and-such will happen," "Someday I'll work at such-and-such a place," etc. In fact, when the *Tokyo Shimbun* article appeared, I thought, "I knew this would happen."

I had imagined for a long while beforehand even the angle I wanted to be photographed from for the accompanying picture. I had an image of myself in my mind of me speaking in the spotlight on a stage long before I was asked to speak at a big event sponsored by *Nikkei Woman*, a Japanese businesswomen's magazine.

Once, on a business trip to the city of Osaka, I stayed in a high-end hotel with a gorgeous lobby. It impressed me greatly. There was a beautiful fountain on the 26th floor, and the manners of the hotel staff were impressive. So at that time I envisioned intensely that someday I would give lessons in a place like that. I recreated the image in my mind over and over again like a mantra.

Then, two years later, an offer came to deliver a lecture in front of 200 people at that very hotel. Posters featuring yours truly appeared as advertisements in the subway trains there. When I first saw them, I felt shivers down my spine.

Method 6: Turn yourself into a luxury brand

These days, many women in their 20's and 30's want to pursue a career as well as find a suitable marriage partner.

A variety of diet books, anti-aging secrets and various other self-improvement seminars and products to help women achieve these goals are flooding the market. I want you to remember, though, that the beauty you can buy easily doesn't last very long.

One day one of the students who was taking my lesson complimented me, "Your jeans are very nice. What brand are they?"

I tried to avoid answering directly, because it was actually a very cheap brand!

If you fully extend your legs, lift your chest and carry yourself nobly, you'll look amazing even if you're not wearing high-end designer clothing. Even in a t-shirt and plain jeans, if you have good posture you'll look terrific. It's because the confidence that comes from within affects your appearance more than the value of the items you wear on the outside. You should prepare your body before you worry about adorning it.

The other day, I was watching a TV program about a businessman whose annual income had just risen by 3 million yen.

The man surrounded himself with luxury goods, and used up all the money he had saved to buy a house on his appearance instead.

He spent nearly ten million yen ($100,000) on designer clothing and several million more on orthodontics and teeth whitening. After changing his appearance, he got positive responses from companies that had refused to deal with him previously. He even received warm welcomes from offices he visited without an appointment. His previously below-par business performance began to rise dramatically. Due to these experiences, he suggested that an "era of appearance" had dawned.

However, while watching this program, I wondered if what he said was really true.

Although it's really none of my business, I started to worry about the businessman. The appealing façade that he got so effortlessly through money is something he will not be able to maintain unless he keeps investing financially in his appearance for the rest of his life. I wonder how practical such an investment would be. Once we depend on a certain thing, it's very difficult to become independent of it. It's very easy to fall into dependence, and such things always have their limits. However, if you develop a lovely posture, practicing until it's second nature, you'll create an exceedingly attractive bodyline that projects a powerful appearance. Also, it costs nothing. Even when you are wearing something cheap, people will never know thanks to the classy atmosphere your excellent posture gives off.

Method 7: Mirror lessons that nourish your "self"

Most of my students have one complex or another about their bodies. People tend to be more inclined to focus on the negatives, rather than try to feel upbeat about something positive. Apparently the smarter you are, the more likely it is you'll have this habit. When do you think most people have the keenest awareness of their bodies? One of these times is when they get sick. Another is when they obsess about negative aspects of their bodies when they stand in front of the mirror. "I've put on weight recently," or "I have more blemishes on my face than before." Our body frequently gets attention only when something bad has happened, not when it's in good condition. Some people say, "Just to be alive now is so wonderful!" but there are few people who really think so. I am one of the few that really do think so!

In my lessons, I often talk about the importance of the

mirror. When in front of the mirror, you must try to see only your good parts. Try to compliment yourself: "I'm beautiful!" "My skin is soft and sleek!"

When you hang a mirror, try to put it in a position where it helps you look as beautiful as possible. I position the mirror where the lighting is just right so I can't see my wrinkles. The color of the mirror frame is white and gold. I also often decorate the area beside the mirror with flowers so that it looks like the mirror of a princess.

At home, I even talk to myself in the mirror! I don't pay attention to the bad aspects of my appearance. I'm able to see my wrinkles as dimples, which I think is far more pleasant. I tell my students that the trick is to look from head to toe. Then I tell them to look themselves over again after backing up one step. Then I say, "Try to look inside yourself." Don't stare at the mirror and say, "I don't like this or that part of my face." Just pull yourself back a step and look at your whole body from head to toe. You'll find that you don't need to worry over every little part or detail so much. When you're able to look at yourself like this, and realize the balance and form of your whole body, you've mastered the technique of seeing yourself one step removed.

Moreover, to see the inside of yourself is to look into the core of your existence. The important thing is to be able to look at yourself in the mirror and say, "I appreciate that I'm healthy today," or "It's wonderful to be alive."

It might be difficult at first, but if you can feel this way you will be empowered to say, "Today I will live life to the fullest!"

As you learn to truly see yourself, little by little you will become fonder of yourself, leading you closer to true happiness. Then your heart will be strong enough to never falter.

When this happens, you can feel comfortable with yourself the way you are. I think that you can only truly accept others once you learn to accept yourself.

Method 8: How to be treated well by others

If I start to tell you about the complexes I used to have, I'm not sure I will be able to stop.

I am 5'9" (175 cm) tall (which is quite tall for a Japanese woman), and before I started Posture Walking, I had a complex about my height.

I always wanted to be a petite, pretty girl.

I have size 10 feet. There is a saying in Japan: "An idiot has big feet, a fool has small feet." Therefore, it's considered best to have average-sized feet. I took the trouble to ride the long distance to school by bicycle when I was in high school, because some boys that I didn't even know teased me about my feet right to my face if I took the train to school. I thought, "I wish I could trim my feet," so many times.

I have apologized to my feet. "I'm sorry I abused you for being yourselves." Now, I always thank them.

I don't think it's necessarily bad to think, "I want to be beautiful and popular," or "I want to be liked by others." It boils down to the fact that you want to be accepted by someone, right? But that means adapting yourself to fit someone else's standards of beauty. If that becomes your goal in life, I think that's a little sad. Wanting to improve yourself is a good thing, but if trying to do so ruins your life, your priorities are in the wrong order.

If you always adapt yourself to others, your body will cry out in opposition, and you run the risk of losing your sense of self.

However, if you are able to break away from this kind of mental pattern, your life will change for the better. To do this, you have to treat yourself more delicately, like a flower. Cherish yourself. If you do so, others will treat you well, too. This is what I've come to realize.

I often talk about "princess time" to my students.

I believe that every woman should try to put aside even a little time to treat themselves like a princess and feel from the bottom of their hearts that they are splendidly beautiful.

When you drink coffee, buy the best coffee beans, use good quality water and indulge. Feel the coffee seep into your body little by little. I think that if you give yourself just ten minutes of this kind of luxurious time each day it will make a big difference in your life.

I also like to show how little luxuries can be an example of a good use of material possessions. It's important to have at least one "luxury object" or item among the things you surround yourself with in your life. It's all right if it is only a small bag or a fountain pen, but you shouldn't compromise on what you really want—even if it's expensive. If you have two hours free time, have lunch at a nice restaurant. Don't strain to get something beyond your reach and don't buy something just to show off to others. In your private, personal space, try to spend some time in elegant leisure.

Just by supplementing your lifestyle with little luxuries, you'll start to see changes. But if you think, "None of this means anything," nothing will change.

If you always make do with cheap things, your heart will be clouded by a cheap mood. If you always wear cheap clothes, the wind will poke through the holes in the fabric and penetrate your heart.

Even still, simply buying brand-name goods cannot substitute for the little luxuries I recommend. What I intend is for you to look for little luxuries that are meaningful.

It's essential to make time to treat yourself like an exquisite flower. By doing this you'll gain the confidence to cherish yourself and the core of your heart will grow strong.

Method 9: Harnessing your mind to create a good "mental posture"

My motto is: "Be happy every day."

When I get up, I feel the sunshine wash over my whole body and I say, "Thank you for the fine weather!"

Then I say, "I'm needed by my students today!" and, "I'm so beautiful today." This gives my body the emotional nutrition it needs.

If you think that you have to try hard and do your best 24/7, the mental effort can overwhelm you. I try to take it step by step by telling myself, "I will spend this hour, this minute, happily."

I travel for work very often, and therefore don't stay in one place for very long. Even so, I never fail to make a little princess time for myself. When I stay in a hotel, even if it only has a small bathroom, I put a few drops of aroma oil into the tub. Even if it's just one night, I buy a flower from a nearby shop to liven up the atmosphere.

I think this is a representation of my mental posture, or stance of my spirit.

Every year I plan a Cinderella Tour.

It aims to provide the opportunity to play princess, something that almost every girl dreams of at least once in her life. The tour went to Italy in 2005, France in 2006, and Austria in 2007.

We all dressed up and behaved like elegant princesses and spent time living in a dream. We had decadent meals and stayed in old castles or first-class hotels. We watched operas from special booth seats.

Every year the tour immediately sells out.

During the tour we are considerate of ourselves and focus on self-love. Everyone is smiling the entire time, and many women say, "This is the first time in my life I've had such a wonderful experience!"

It's a wonderful tour with the power to drastically change people's view of life.

Since autumn of 2006, I've also offered a domestic Japanese tour. Some of the activities and topics we focus on are: "Get a haircut while surrounded by nature!" and "Bare your heart and mind." The aim for these activities is to reset your body and mind, in effect going back to nature. We call it the

Natural Tour.

I think the more you experience pleasure in every part of your being, the more you can honestly say to yourself, "I'm happy." Happy experiences will turn into happy memories that stay with you forever.

I believe those are the building blocks to leading a happier life.

Method 10:
The internal balance needed to accept others

I'm sure people have heard the terms "narcissist" or "self-obsessed."

When I talk about focusing on the self, some people misinterpret my meaning. What I intend to convey is my singular dedication to not doing things half-heartedly. It's completely opposite to the notions of "I only care about my own needs," or "I don't have to think about other people or what they want."

What I mean is that we can start to care about others only once we learn to accept ourselves. After I started Posture Walking, I found time to focus just on myself, thereby relieving some of the pressures in my life.

Some others that I became acquainted with through my children's school sometimes ask, "Walking classes sound really good. But is starting such a thing at this stage of my life really going to make a difference?"

If I had heard these kinds of criticisms when I had just started teaching, I'm sure I would have panicked. However, the pleasure of walking properly and my gratitude towards my life is very secure now. My way of life has become very simple. I realize that there's no need to show off. I lost the urge to compete with others, preferring instead to wish for their happiness. Everyone is capable of such feelings.

I feel love for myself from the bottom of my heart.

When we focus on and give love to ourselves, we're able to cherish others as well. It's due to this realization that I could become happier that I'm truly happy now.

I think balance is important in everything. Feeling the desire to be someone special or to be better than others often leads us to negate ourselves or hurt other people. The "I want to be special" way of thinking is a short-sighted mindset focusing on the future that denies your here and now, while also threatening your body's balance.

The body instinctively tries to balance itself. The pelvis, spine, neck and head are all connected, so if my pelvis is twisted, my spine will be twisted as well. Everything is connected in our body.

I think it's best to use common sense and be natural, not necessarily "special." When it comes to beauty, the best kind is not beauty that makes others nervous, but beauty that makes others feel relaxed and happy. A natural beauty that shines out from inside. It is not the kind of beauty that competes with others but the kind that causes others to sympathize with you.

Your true beauty exists in a form that only you can possess.

If you have good balance, you look stable. That makes others feel safe around you. People feel at ease when dealing with someone whose body and mind are both balanced.

I believe that when we have trained our bodies to move gracefully, we're able to have a harmonious, balanced life amid society.

So let's walk with our chests high and our feet firmly on the ground. The first steps towards a positive life are proper posture and graceful walking.

Method 11: Which way is your life's sail set?

When I visited an old castle in Loire, France, I took a walk through the garden. The castle was located in a big forest. Small wild violets were in full bloom and the softly rotting leaves underfoot made me feel so comfortable.

"Wow, I'm walking on the earth. I feel the warmth of the earth."

While I was thinking along these lines, a question suddenly popped up.

"Why do we have toes?"

These kinds of thoughts are my occupational obsession. There are animals that can grip onto the trunks of trees with their feet. Do we use our feet at maximum efficiency? I moved and wriggled my toes in many ways. While I was doing this, I laughed at myself for bothering to care about such a strange, minor thing.

"If I push off the ground with only my toes, will I engage my stomach muscles because my body will lean forward? Aha! If I use the entire sole of my foot I can feel my abs working!"

I listened to my body for a full 24 hours. Every part of my body was "thinking" about walking.

"How can I 'switch on' my muscles and get them to engage more quickly? Can I lose weight by using my muscles naturally?"

At that time I realized the importance of using your toes properly.

Some time later, I was studying with Dr. Garrick, who is a well-known orthopedic surgeon, at a hospital in San Francisco. There I discovered a book that described the superficial back line. The book had descriptions and pictures of all the body's muscles. By reading through this, I learned that the muscles on the back of the body are interconnected: from the soles of the feet through the posterior, back muscles, back of the neck and up to the forehead.

There'd been quite a few students who exclaimed, "The wrinkles disappeared from my forehead once I started Posture Walking!" but until I read about the superficial back line, I didn't have any clear scientific explanation for why this was happening. Once I figured it out, everything fell into place.

The method of Posture Walking, where we use the muscles in our toes, developed throughout my daily experiments and through my teaching experiences.

I made all these little discoveries on my own, gleaned from what my body was telling me. If this sounds odd, you have my permission to not take me seriously. Still, I have unshakable confidence in myself.

My body is living evidence that proves the positive effects of Posture Walking. The core of every walking method is similar by nature. However, the forms and expressions differ. My Posture Walking method is the expression of my way of living.

It has been 9 years since I first began Posture Walking. I

taught my first class 7 years ago. I started with 8 students. I now have over 60,000.

However, when I look back, it seems like it all happened in a flash. I didn't have time to pause and reflect on everything that was happening as it occurred. I just did my very best, trying to be a great teacher one class at a time. I, who used to be your average full-time housewife, was reborn after discovering Posture Walking. Now I have a completely different life. I am walking through my second life.

I've come to think that I'm simply borrowing my body from a higher power, and that I'm not really of this world! I don't want to go into a strange theory of the spirit, but in any case, the way I now live my life suits me just fine.

So the wheels of my life have been set into motion. I'll occasionally gently realign the rudder, but I think I succeed just by understanding which direction my sail should be set to catch the wind.

Before now, I tried groping about blindly, flailing one direction then shifting to another. But since learning how to move my body properly, I am now able to turn my sail 360 degrees. This allows me to lock in on the currents or frequencies as they change according to the delicate nuances of the seasons.

Without straining at all, I'm able to realign myself in a

way that benefits me the most.

I'm very lucky to have developed this kind of sensitivity after turning 40. Absolutely anyone, no matter how old, has the ability to set their sail to catch the wind that suits them best. So be honest with yourself and respectful of your body.

Everyone has a body, and before long you'll see that that connects you to everyone in the world. You'll begin to cherish others in the same way you cherish yourself.

There are infinite possibilities in your own body.

CHAPTER 3

The Body Method

Method 1: How walking can remove forehead wrinkles and tone your buttocks

Let me introduce the basics of Posture Walking

This method of walking gives you an outstanding butt-lifting effect by doing nothing other than walking effectively. This is done by placing your balance on your heels and using the muscles in your back. While doing this, keep the muscles in the front of your body relaxed.

It's a little difficult at first. If you pay too much attention to particular muscles, you'll tense up.

You want to be at the point where the muscles down your back are engaged, while the muscles in your front are relaxed. When I figured out the secret of this muscle-use method, I became more comfortable and lost a lot of tension.

If you walk with your muscles engaged like this, you'll have greater energy, even if you walk for a long while. At the same time, you'll gain very good muscle tone down the back of your body, making you look elegant and beautiful.

I think this method of walking is revolutionary. Right now, I'm in the process of applying for a patent on it!

As I mentioned before, the muscles in the toes are linked to the head and forehead through the muscles along the back of the body.

A lot of my students say, "I lost wrinkles from my forehead thanks to Posture Walking." My forehead is also wrinkle-free.

To enhance the effect, when you move your legs as you walk, roll each foot along the ground from heel to toe. I call this "rolling." Just before lifting your foot off the ground at the end of each pace, stretch your toes out and push off.

The wrinkles on your face are caused by slack skin on your head. So when you walk, if you make it a habit to stretch your toes, the muscles of your forehead will strengthen and the skin between your eyebrows will tighten!

Method 2:
Walking effectively to activate your Positivity Switch

A while ago, I had a female student who was 72 years old.

One day she said to me, "I've wanted to learn something

new, but everything seemed too difficult for me. It's very hard for me to take the first step. But I thought Posture Walking might be easy enough to try."

So she started taking classes.

This woman couldn't travel far due to an incontinence problem that she had. Even still, she managed to attend every one of my lessons, commenting eagerly, "I'm so happy to be able to walk with young people." However, while learning how to walk properly, she gradually gained strength in her abdominal muscles. After several weeks she told me, "I've gotten stronger and more confident, so I'm taking a trip to Italy with my husband." I was so happy for her.

When I see the effect my teaching has on others, I'm very happy. Seeing each of my students find joy is the best thing in my life.

One night, I congregated with my students in the flashy Ginza district of Tokyo so that we could all practice walking together. Everyone strode together, showing off what our practice had achieved.

Naturally, we stood out in the crowd. Men sharing after-work drinks watched our group pass by. We heard some of them exclaim, "Wow!" They might have just been mocking us, but some tried to follow us around. We all laughed out loud and beamed with joy. "It's so amazing we can have this much fun just by walking!" "Posture Walking makes me feel so happy!" Walking, especially when done properly, is very fun. We get used to taking a train or a car, and end up feeling like walking for any distance is a bother or a chore.

People have forgotten the huge advantages and benefits that come from proper walking.

Walking hump-backed, walking without engaging your upper body or walking with arm and leg movements that are unbalanced—there are many ways to walk incorrectly. These things occur when the body is not properly balanced. It's as if the brain's signals aren't reaching the limbs.

However, when someone walks beautifully, you can see that they have excellent awareness and control over their body's use.

I once had a student who started off quite badly. Her muscles were weak and she hated to walk very far until she began taking lessons. She had suffered from eczema since she was little. She then developed sciatica in her 20's, leaving her in a poor physical condition.

When she first came to take lessons, she was already married. She was extremely pigeon-toed and she walked with her back slumped over. This caused her to tire easily. It seemed to be a challenge to even draw breath.

She said that her husband had encouraged her to take

walking lessons, even though she tended to keep herself shut up in the house. She took his advice and started to take lessons.

Over the course of a year of lessons, her manner of walking and posture changed, and she grew strong enough to be able to walk for a long time. She was then able to find the joy of walking. She enjoyed going out for walks or to shop. When she was able to see walking as a positive thing, her outlook on life brightened. Miraculously, she recovered from her eczema completely. This was the most surprising development. What's more, she later became pregnant. She gave birth to a fine, healthy baby.

"I figured I was too weak to ever hope for a baby," she said. "But thanks to you, I now have a healthy baby." She was so happy. She was a garrulous and attractive mother and was like a different person compared to how she used to be.

The word "walk" or "step" is often used as a metaphor for the progress one makes in life. This student's experience reflects this meaning well, don't you think?

Getting rid of your bad habits and learning proper body use will unleash the energy you have always had within your own body. People who walk while focusing on positivity— feeling happy, fun, pleasant—will discover that life holds many treasures. Beginning to walk properly is akin to creating your life anew. Walking can reveal your true potential.

Method 3: The beauty of unaffected walking

While losing weight and getting into shape is a pleasant side effect of walking properly, it's still important to focus on a "normal" seeming walking method that can be used even when you're out in public.

You might think that makes it seem like my technique is nothing special at all. But let me explain. By "normal" I mean a way of walking that is unaffected and free from bad habits. It's actually harder than it looks.

Let's look at a model walking on a runway, for example. That's called "catwalking." It's a special method intended to show off the designs of the clothing (and the beauty of the model). It's a very flashy type of walking.

My method is of a different sort. It's a type of walking we can use in our daily lives. I think walking that enhances the balance between your body and mind is truly beautiful walking.

If you can free yourself from your bad habits, you'll discover your own beauty. My method of walking may not seem particularly outstanding or revolutionary on the outside, but it does produce an effect that brings out your inner beauty, that gives you a positive aura.

Moreover, this way of walking that I strive for still falls in the category of "everyday walking."

Method 4: How to correct your walking habits

During lessons, I ask my students to walk from one side of the studio to the other while I videotape them.

Naturally, this makes everybody tense, and their movements become more awkward. This highlights and accentuates their bad habits. Students can then see and understand their bad habits by watching themselves in the video.

One of the good points about doing this in the classroom is that there's more than one person watching objectively. All of the students watch together. "Your movement has changed!" "You look completely different!" People burst into applause. This encourages the students and makes them feel eager to continue on to the next step.

"I've straightened my posture. I feel good." "I can move very well!" The more positive people feel about their progress, the more progress they make.

By losing your rigidity, stiffness and bad habits, your way of walking will be far more elegant and attractive than it was before. If you work on this step by step, you will notice a positive change.

However, not everything can change dramatically overnight. I've noticed that it usually takes around two years before you notice major changes, both physical and mental.

If you continually think, "I must walk beautifully," "I must fix my posture," "I must lose weight," and have feelings of duty to these "musts" then you'll have a tough time. It's important to keep thinking positively all the time, rather than just "making an effort," "enduring" or "bearing it."

"Just by lifting my chest and raising up my face, I noticed for the first time the beauty of the sky, even though I was walking the same route I always take." My students often send me these kinds of glowing letters and e-mails.

"I'll try to hold my face up a little more than usual today." "I'll try to keep my arms towards my back as I walk." Start by trying these easy, simple things to train your body. The muscle memory will spread until each cell in your body will realign itself to a new method of walking.

I want you to approach your feelings the same way. Don't compare yourself to others. Don't be negative, thinking, "I can't do this or that." Do what you can without beating yourself up.

Start with one small adjustment. If done purposefully, you'll turn on the positivity switch. This is because every part of your body is connected to everything else. Finding one pleasure will lead you to more pleasant discoveries. It creates a domino effect of positivity.

Method 5:
The influence of good posture on your figure

Whether you have a good figure or not depends a great deal on your posture.

If you keep your body well balanced, you'll look extremely attractive regardless of how tall, short, heavy or thin you are.

If a tall person does not have confidence because of their height and walk with a hunched back, they will spoil their fine figure.

I used to be one such person.

On the other hand, short people tend to wish they were taller.

The important thing is not to try and be taller but to use your body as fully as possible. Then, regardless of your height, you'll be attractive.

If you use your body efficiently, avoid pushing yourself unreasonably or comparing yourself negatively to others, you can make the most of the body that you have now.

To develop that kind of perspective is important. People feel envious of others if they're not pleased with their own body. Once you have started to understand proper body use, you'll have no time to worry over complexes.

The first part of standing properly is to place your feet firmly on the ground. You can feel energy coming up through you, just from feeling your feet against the ground. Focus on the feeling of being recharged by the earth.

When I say, "Stand straight with good posture," many people stick out their chests and throw their backs out of kilt. This is incorrect. Don't put extra pressure on your body. If you do, you'll tire easily.

Picture the core of your body. Then hold the image of directly aligning your head with your heels. This will make your quads, abs and glutes much stronger.

Method 6: Work on appropriate body language

When I hold training seminars for companies, I often talk about posture. A person with good posture not only looks good, but also affects the surrounding atmosphere in a positive way. In contrast, a person with poor posture can make the surrounding atmosphere seem distasteful, and bad posture worsens one's attitude and undermines morale. Eventually the general attitude of the company sours, and the company's products are negatively affected as well.

Walk beautifully and behave beautifully. This makes the atmosphere around you pleasant. If the company has a lot of positive staff members, the company's brand and image will improve.

This is something that cannot be bought with money, yet is incredibly valuable.

As soon as a customer enters a store, they will have an impression of the place based on the general mood or atmosphere of the place or its staff.

For example, if the staff members have good posture, even without saying anything, the customer will feel satisfied by the way they're welcomed. It's another form of nonverbal communication.

The most important things at the initial stage of welcoming a customer are posture, pleasant facial expression and eye contact.

All employees, even if they are trainees, should carry themselves well while keeping in mind that every one of them represents the company and the brand.

A smile can reduce the distance between people and facilitate communication. Eye contact shows that you are capable of accepting the other person, as well as showing that you have confidence. From that point on your confidence emanates from your eyes. Trust emanates from your chest. The degree of confidence you inspire is directly related to your posture.

The way the staff handles the products or merchandise is also a form of nonverbal communication. If the staff member's fingers are neatly arranged and give off a sense of politeness and care, the customers will feel they are being treated respectfully as well.

When you pick up the phone or open your bag, use your hands gracefully and with care. When you sit, lay your hands one on top of the other and put your knees and toes together. With these movements, a woman's beauty really shines.

It's important to be aware of the appropriateness of your body language.

Method 7: Overcoming complexes about your legs

Whether we're standing or walking, our legs have the all-important role of supporting our bodies. Unfortunately, there's probably only a small percentage of people that are satisfied enough with their legs to be able to think, "I have great legs." It seems that most people have varying complaints about their legs. They're too fat, too short, too hairy, etc.

In fact, I used to be one of the many who had major worries about my legs. I was bow-legged. When I was younger, my right leg curved outwards. This caused me to develop a complex and I avoided wearing short skirts.

But after discovering Posture Walking and learning

how to carry my legs and balance my posture the complex disappeared quickly. Without getting an operation to remedy my bowlegs, my legs look straight, even in photos.

During my lessons, I have my students look at my legs in order to convince them that I am in fact bow-legged. It's impossible to cure bowlegs or knock-knees or totally alter the shape of your legs through walking alone. However, it's easy to disguise such problems by correcting posture, alignment and walking method.

When I say, "We can cheat! It's the same thing as wearing makeup!" the students that have these kinds of worries all smile with relief.

If your problems cease to bother you, your complexes will vanish. The "problem" seems less worrisome when the complex disappears, even if the shape of your legs has not changed at all.

Method 8: Respect your legs!

When I have a lesson, I always tell my students things like, "Take good care of your legs for the rest of your life. It's a longer commitment than marriage! If you take good care of your legs, they'll never betray you."

I always compliment my own legs after my walking lessons. Giving your legs a compliment is like giving them a magical treat. Such words nourish the nerves in your legs. Soon the nerves are strengthening your veins and increasing blood flow. This encourages your body to build muscle.

A beautiful body can be created by your consciousness as well. People often say that if you talk to your plants, they'll grow faster. My idea is similar to this concept. With only a few words of encouragement, our body reacts like a plant reacts to sunlight or rain.

This kind of phenomenon can be compared to mother's milk. A mother won't produce milk unless the baby needs it, and the more a baby wants, the more milk comes out. However, if a baby doesn't nurse, nothing comes out.

It's the same with our bodies. The more affection we give our bodies, the more positively our bodies will react. Every part of your body will cry out, "Life, more life!"

Method 9: How to walk beautifully in high heels

Depending on the TPO (Time, Place, Occasion), I sometimes wear high heels.

You must remember though that in the case of high heels, the body's center of gravity tends to pitch forward. This makes it difficult to put weight on your heels. In addition, if you wear heels for a long time, they will gradually cause your toes to become twisted or even disfigured. Therefore it's important to adjust the way you stand and walk when wearing heels. When standing, engage your abdominals and lift up your chest so that your toes don't take the entire burden. The use of your abs is the key.

If you can keep your pelvis facing straight forward, tucking the tailbone slightly, you can maintain a natural posture. In heels the lower back tends to curve inward, the pelvis tilts forward and the knees stay in flexion, which can cause the feet to swell.

It might seem sexy for young women to push their hips out while wearing heels, but at the very least, it doesn't make them look very smart.

Adult women should wear high heels more intelligently.

Keep your knees moving directly from back to front in smooth swings, imagining a line from the heels, through the knees, and up to the body. Don't let the knees jut out to the sides.

What is even sexier is when the kneecap of the back leg comes forward and passes the kneecap of the front leg and they just barely graze each other as they cross.

From there the calf and ankle of the moving leg cross the standing leg's calf and ankle. It's very sexy.

In high heels, you can't kick off the ground like you can in sneakers, so keep your knee straight as you bring each leg forward.

When buying high heels, try to find a pair with wide heels. This makes it easier to put some weight on the heels, easing the strain on your toes.

Method 10: Kimiko's "Walking Pilates"

One of the major reasons I started walking lessons at age 36 was the fact that I had a very hard time recovering my figure after the birth of my second son. However, as I started walking, my body started to change so much that it seemed like I had gotten full-body cosmetic surgery. My waist became inches thinner and even my height increased—I grew one inch taller.

When it comes to Posture Walking, I have witnessed the benefits firsthand.

Just from walking, my figure changed and I started to feel more positive. It transformed my life completely.

How can something as simple as walking change your life so much?

Mr. Naokata Ishii, an expert in muscle physiology and a well-known writer, accepted my request for me to interview him for one of my earlier books. He had this to say:

"What I recommend most for the common person to do without going to too much trouble to lose weight while maintaining elegance, is to train the psoas major. This is very easy to do. Simply walk with proper posture, with your back straight. That's it."

If you walk beautifully, you'll actually be training your muscles. This leads to a lifting of the bust, refining of the hips, slimming of the waist, and the slimming down of your legs.

The psoas major is an important muscle used in walking. It's one of the hip flexor muscles and is situated deep in the core of the body. It starts at the inside of the femur, comes forward, up and over the pelvis then heads back again, attaching to the base of the spine. It's said that muscle training can't strengthen the psoas major alone, but walking properly is very beneficial. When I first heard this I was impressed. Since then I've become very interested in anatomy and physiology, and I have started to study scientific approaches to walking as well.

The method of posture walking is an original idea that was born from my personal experience. The scientific aspects are currently being tested.

One expert that interprets walking in the context of the body-mind connection is Dr. Junya Takeda, the director of Takeda Sports and Nutrition Clinic, who is well known as the first person in Japan to establish a medical treatment institution that includes a Pilates studio.

"As walking is a continuous exercise, the muscles

used are constantly being stimulated. The activity of brain neurotransmitters is elevated. We can balance the mind while achieving moderate stimulation to the visual and balance receptors in the brain. Kimiko's posture walking method, also referred to as 'walking Pilates,' is an effective health preserving measure that links directly to anti-aging."

Walking has many scientifically based effects on the body as well as the mind.

Method 11: How the mind is navigated by the body

Many people think it's difficult to control emotions and feelings, but I think it's something that can be mastered with practice.

If we can develop control over our bodies, we can control our minds as well. If you can control your manner of walking, you can take conscious control of your movement to a considerably degree. I think the body and mind are one, or at least very intimately connected.

I want to introduce a very impressive student I had as an example. This student would hyperventilate and panic whenever she rode a train or was in a cramped, crowded space. She became agoraphobic so she shut herself up in her home and spent most of her time sleeping. This lasted for a year and a half.

One day she started taking walking lessons. As she progressed, her mind and body began to recover as she became more positive. One thing she told me that I was particularly impressed by was that after she went back to her old job, she broke-down and cried one day when things weren't going well. To try and calm herself down, she started to walk as I had taught her with her chest forward and lifted. This simple exercise allowed her to regain her confidence and positivity.

She also practiced my recommended exercise of looking into a mirror and praising herself every day.

"After I realized I could love myself, the reaction of other people towards me changed miraculously," she said.

Since she started Posture Walking, her figure, which proved resistant to dieting, started to change. Moreover, her panic attacks ceased.

I have no intention of trying to sell a snake-oil "mental disease can be mended by walking" concept. What I want to do is explain that our body has infinite possibilities that lie dormant. Will power and positivity are very powerful things.

There will be big differences in your life depending on whether you develop your body into something limitless, or whether you limit and restrict your body's capabilities and possibilities.

If more people poured love into and showed appreciation for their bodies, a tremendous power would well up in their minds, empower their way of living and create positive change in the world.

Posture Lessons

The characteristics of Posture Walking

The great thing about my original method of Posture Walking is that it can be done whenever, wherever, and by anyone. It's very practical.

The distortions that accumulate within our bodies throughout our daily lives gradually disappear just by walking properly, whether you're young or not. It allows us to refresh both our minds and bodies.

Walking beautifully allows you to get your life back.

Walking

This way of walking beautifully has you keeping your head directly in line with your heels and pelvis. Keep most of your weight towards the back of your body as you walk.

Points:

1. Lead with your back. Keep your weight balanced

towards the back of your body and initiate walking from your back.

2. With each step roll from your heel onto your toes. Stretch out your toes as you push off the ground.

3. Be conscious of all the muscles along your back.

4. When swinging your arms, make sure your hands extend beyond the back of your body.

Point 1: Lead with your back

Begin by standing with good posture. Then imagine that a big hand is pushing the middle of your back. If you're female, leave a space the size of a fist between your big toes and rotate your heels about one inch inwards. Begin walking, placing each heel on an imaginary straight line one after the other. Stretch each leg out straight as it moves forward.

Imagine the entire lower half of your body—starting at your navel—is part of your legs. Extend your knees and take broad steps.

Keep your center of gravity balanced towards your back and lead with your back. While you are doing this, it's important to relax the front of your body.

Point 2: Rolling

The importance of rolling (the movement from your heel

to toes) can't be emphasized enough. When one of your legs is moving forward into the next step, keep your weight on the other leg. Land on your heel and roll your weight along your foot towards your toes. When your back leg pushes off the ground, use your toes, stretching them out fully.

If you master this rolling technique, you'll notice various positive effects.

By rolling along your foot in this way, the balls of your feet are stimulated (which are connected to the heart, according to reflexology), which leads to improved blood circulation while reducing swelling.

Rolling is a fundamental aspect of Posture Walking. Land each step slightly on the outer edge of the heel, press the entire bottom of your foot into the ground and smoothly send your body's weight forward into the next step.

Before landing on the heel, your knee should straighten. As you take each step you'll feel like you're in touch with the earth.

Realizing how each step connects you to the earth will make you feel joyful. You might even experience a warm feeling like rubbing a whale's belly. (I've never actually rubbed one myself, though.)

Moreover, stretching out your toes as you walk helps remove wrinkles from your forehead. This is because the muscles in your toes are connected to all the muscles along the back, up to the muscles on the back of the head, which in turn connect to the forehead. However, if you place too much weight on the outside of your feet (walking "duck-toed") you'll put pressure on the second toe and possibly cause bunions. If you go too far the other way and walk pigeon-toed, all of your weight will fall onto your pinkie toes and it becomes difficult to push off the ground with any force.

Picture a line extending straight from the sole of your foot right to the center of the earth. This line also extends from the head straight to the heavens. Our bodies fit perfectly along the axis between heaven and earth.

The trick of rolling is to kick off the ground as if your foot is sinking into it. This stabilizes your pelvis. Work to master this rolling technique.

Point 3:
Keep your back foot on the ground for as long as possible

Before pushing off the ground with your back foot, wait until the last possible moment, leaving your foot on the ground as long as possible. Pay attention to your buttocks, thighs, knees and calves.

If the back of your knee is stretched out comfortably, your hip flexors should be fully stretched, and the bottom part of your glutes and hamstrings should be engaged. This will help your buttocks to become firmer and more lifted.

Stretch your front leg out forward while maintaining an imaginary vertical line through the length of your upper body.

Point 4: Arms

If your arms dangle, or if they swing in random, scattered directions, you'll spoil your good posture. When your arms swing towards your back, make sure they move further past your body than they do when they swing forward. In order to swing your arms elegantly, don't open them out too far to the sides; think of pulling them in towards the center of your back. Keep your fingers relaxed without scrunching them up or adding tension.

If you master this arm movement method, you'll tighten up your triceps simply by moving elegantly. Moreover, this method is very effective in tightening any flab on your back. Stretch out through your fingers and be conscious of your shoulder blades alternately folding inwards and engaging the back muscles. This will tone the muscles between the shoulder blades. From now on focus on creating sexy "back cleavage."

During Posture Walking, be sure to stretch out your arms and legs when they move towards your back. It really looks great.

Stretch out your knees!

Stretch out your arms!

But if you think too much about it you'll look like a stiff robot when you walk, so just focus on this point for a moment. If you can find the proper placement even when standing still, your way of walking will become livelier and very stylish.

With this method you're using your muscles properly, so you can also expect to get into better shape.

And that feels pretty good, too!

With proper body use, your muscles all work in harmony to create beautiful body lines.

Become aware of the movements of your shoulder blades and straighten your arms as they swing back. Match your arm swing to the rhythm of your gait and stretch your arms out smoothly.

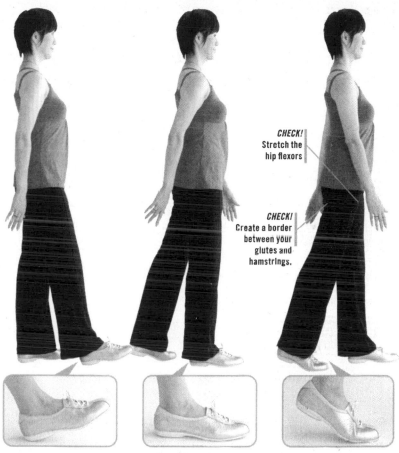

CHECK!
Stretch the
hip flexors

CHECK!
Create a border
between your
glutes and
hamstrings.

With your center of
gravity held above your
back heel, place your
front heel towards the
center of your body and
step forward.

When you transfer your
weight from the back
leg to the front, roll
through your back foot.
At the end, stretch out
your back knee.

Once your center of
gravity is above your
front heel, stretch out
your front knee. Hold
your torso straight.

Keep your head over your heels.

Maintain your center of gravity towards your back when you walk. Your heels, buttocks, shoulder blades and back of your head should all be aligned.

Rotate your heel slightly inwards.

Place your heel towards the middle of your body with each step. Stretch out both knees when you transfer your weight from the back leg to the front.

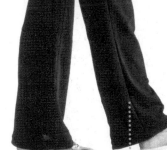

POINT 1

POINT 2

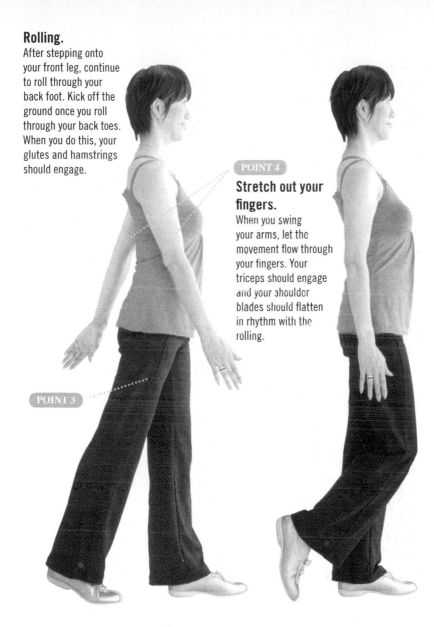

Rolling.

After stepping onto your front leg, continue to roll through your back foot. Kick off the ground once you roll through your back toes. When you do this, your glutes and hamstrings should engage.

POINT 4

Stretch out your fingers.

When you swing your arms, let the movement flow through your fingers. Your triceps should engage and your shoulder blades should flatten in rhythm with the rolling.

POINT 3

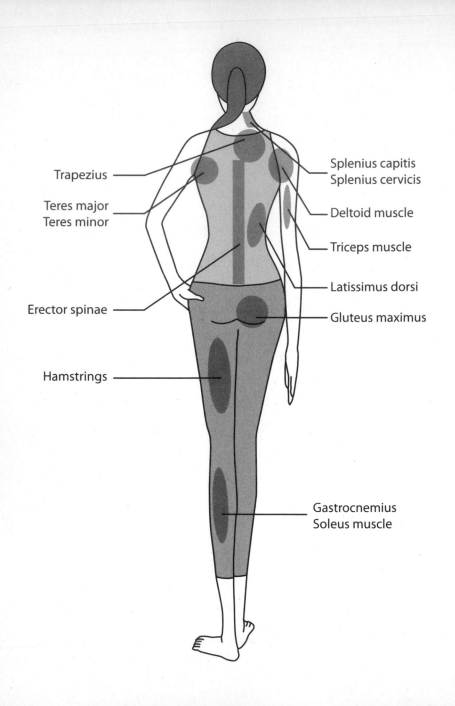

Trapezius

Teres major
Teres minor

Erector spinae

Hamstrings

Splenius capitis
Splenius cervicis

Deltoid muscle

Triceps muscle

Latissimus dorsi

Gluteus maximus

Gastrocnemius
Soleus muscle

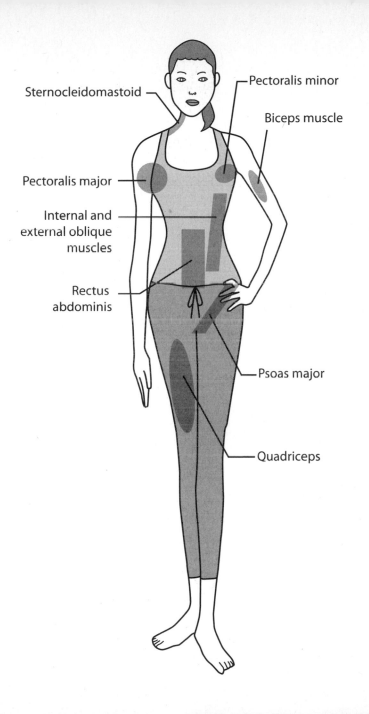

Sternocleidomastoid

Pectoralis minor

Biceps muscle

Pectoralis major

Internal and external oblique muscles

Rectus abdominis

Psoas major

Quadriceps

Psoas Muscle

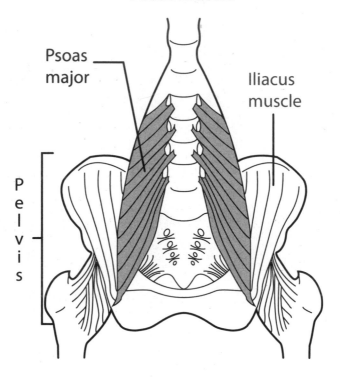

Psoas major

Iliacus muscle

Pelvis

EXERCISES

Core Muscle Training

• Stand on one leg with your knee perfectly straight. Do reps of one to three minutes per leg.

• Lying down facing upward, cross both arms over your chest, press your hips and lower back into the floor and sit up. Using your abdominals slowly raise your upper torso and head, then lay back down even more slowly. Curve your back into a "C" during each rep. Do ten repetitions each morning.

This exercise is very helpful in protecting your lower back. Dr. Garrick taught me this technique. In my own personal experience, my body became much stronger in just three days.

Heaven-Human-Earth Exercise

Slowly raise both arms while turning at the wrists and shoulders so your palms constantly face toward the ceiling.

End with both arms straight up in a "hooray" pose with

your palms facing upwards.

You've done this exercise perfectly if you can keep your wrists at such an angle while keeping your elbows straight!

Picture a line of muscles tightening starting below the shoulders, travelling diagonally across your back to the opposite leg. This exercise beautifully trims the waist.

I gave it this name because you stand straight between the heavens and the earth. It feels good! You can't have good posture if your shoulders are stiff. This is a wonderful exercise to loosen the muscles in the shoulders as well as improve waist definition.

Other Useful Tips

• Do ankle rotations. Ten rotations, slowly, first clockwise, then counter-clockwise.

• Spread and relax your toes. Try playing rock-paper-scissors with your toes.

• Give your lower legs a thorough massage. Start with one toe at a time. Then work the base of each toe followed by the ankles (inside and outside), heels then calves.

• Stretch your hamstrings. Stand with your legs wide apart and with your back straight extend your upper body forward. Keep the tips of your toes pointing forward and your chin should aim for your toes. Do all moves slowly and you should feel a good stretch all along the backs of your legs. Relax; don't overdo it.

Proper Alignment While Standing

Let's work on proper standing posture. Picture your body in your mind. Place your head back to its proper position on top of your spine. I think the reason people get hunchbacked is because of poor head position. When writing or texting or using a computer, you're almost always slouching forward as both shoulders droop forward and the spine curves and your chest caves in. When trying to improve posture without taking the position of the head into consideration, people tend to overcompensate and bend their spine back too far. This causes them to tire because they're clenching the muscles in the shoulders. However, if you think about restoring your head back to the proper position above the spine, your shoulder blades will naturally fall back, and you'll have straight and beautiful posture.

Because our heads are quite heavy, if you place it forward your spine will bend and your shoulders will curve in, compensating for the unbalanced weight. If you focus on lifting up your torso and opening up your chest, the trunk of your body will become more balanced and steady. If you maintain that alignment when you walk, you'll be able to keep your beautiful posture. Maintain the proper alignment of your head for maximum stability.

A beautiful posture depends on the position of the head and the angle of the pelvis. Imagine placing the weight of your head onto your heels, keeping your pelvis slightly tucked, facing straight forward.

Even if your pelvis tends to turn out ("cheerleader rear"), try to tuck the pelvis while leaving a little curve in the spine. Many people who wear high heels often develop a posterior that juts out.

Now then, let's walk, leading with our backs.

After repositioning your head on top of your spine, be sure to maintain that position when you walk. Many people tend to lead with their heads once they start walking. This happens especially if you're in a hurry. Nevertheless, it's important to quickly regain self-control and walk coolly and proudly, like you're the CEO of your own company.

Simply by realigning your posture when you walk, you work the gluteus maximus muscles. A tightened, toned body starts with proper alignment of your head.

This is also true of your posture when seated. The only difference is your legs are bent while sitting. But try and maintain the same sense of alignment.

Keeping your back straight will change the atmosphere around you, giving off a very fresh and invigorating impression.

Keep the front of your body relaxed when you walk. If you clench your leg muscles when stepping forward, your knee will straighten sharply and look robotic. If you focus instead on shifting your center of gravity with each step by pushing off the ground and catching your weight on the fore leg, it lightens your gait and your legs move more naturally. The knee of the leg moving forward will bend smoothly and naturally. When your foot hits the ground, straighten your knee.

Extend your leg out forward. Don't let your knees drift out to the side when you step.

Don't forget to roll along the soles of your feet. The center of gravity moves from the heel along the foot to the toes. Land on your heel first. This is a key point in toning the glutes.

1. Raise the foot going forward slightly.

2. Push off the ground from the ball of your rear foot. Straighten your back knee.

3. Catch your body on your front foot as it moves forward.

Now walk repeating this process in a steady fashion, imagining that each step connects you to the Earth. Roll your feet like they're the base of a rocking chair.

Stretch out your fingers, move your center of gravity forward and straighten your back knee so the backside of your body creates an elegant, straight line. These adjustments will lead to greater muscle tone all over.

Bounce back after each step, each time lifting your body up. Add a bounce to your step!

If you use your legs in this manner you're engaging in a splendid exercise that works your entire body.

In order to use the rolling technique properly, as mentioned, the position of your head is very important.

If you can shift your center of gravity towards your back, the soles of your feet will firmly carry your body's weight. Each step will carry all the way across the bottoms of your feet to the base of your toes. The last step of rolling is the toes pushing off the ground.

The force going downwards into the ground pushes the body upwards.

If your head droops forward you carry your weight onto your toes, and you won't engage the muscles along the backs of your legs or buttocks.

This is the most important aspect of Posture Walking. I discovered that using your legs in this manner is a naturally effective way to shape up your body (as well as improve your figure overall).

I'm not saying you can't make any progress without using the rolling technique. You can still walk even if your head is pushed forward and you're stooped over. However, it's very likely you're not engaging your glutes or properly using your ankles.

But if you are going to walk, doesn't it make sense to do so in a way that firms the muscles, looks graceful, and creates an attractive body line? In other words, this is a luxurious way of moving.

In the back side of your legs are the accelerator muscles (glutes, hamstrings and calves). These are the muscles that mainly work to move your body forward. On the other side, in the front of your legs, are the "brake" muscles. When taking a step it is easy to apply power here.

If you use energy from your accelerator muscles your body will smoothly push forward. If you engage the muscles in the backs of your legs the position of your head will stay back. However, don't push your stomach out when you walk. That could lead to lower back pain.

Another great aspect of this walking technique is that it helps you smile. Isn't it hard to smile when your face is drooping down?

Bounce your weight off the ground. Bring your head up and flip on the positivity switch.

The power of a smile starts with your body. Walking with a straight back is like smiling with your whole body.

The importance of rolling

It was at a shopping promenade in a tony part of San Francisco where there were many beautiful women walking around.

There I saw a group of well-dressed older women sitting around talking and noticed they all had something in common. Despite the fact their style was impeccable, after they finished chatting and one stood up and started walking, I realized how old she was. How did she walk? Slowly, with her toes hitting the ground first, and then lifting the heel of her back foot when stepping off.

It looked like the way a cat walks, but those were heavy steps.

On top of that, she didn't lift her feet very high off the ground, so she might stumble and fall on something as small as a pebble. With this way of walking the knees are not extended straight. This is typical of the elderly. The muscles appear to be weak. This is how I came to realize the importance of rolling if you want to walk elegantly.

When I look at how elderly people (or even ambitionless young people) walk I notice that almost none of them use rolling. They walk flat-footed. This could lead to degeneration of both the body and the spirit.

Even without any special insight, you can see they don't seem cheerful.

"Are you not feeling well?"

"Are you in a bad mood?"

I think posture has a lot to do with one's mood.

Also I have seen very overweight people "waddle" when they walk. They rock from left to right, using their excess weight like a pendulum and not using the muscles in their legs, let alone rolling.

Common errors in the beginning

At first it's difficult to find the rhythm and balance needed while also straightening the back leg. Unconsciously the head shifts forward and droops down. Without stretching out the hip flexors, the next step is taken before the knees are suitably straightened. Too much tension forms in the upper body causing the torso to fall forward. This also means the center of gravity is too far forward, putting a burden on the knees. Footfalls get louder.

Keep the head towards the back, on top of the spine. Keep your neck gently straight, like a king or queen.

It's easy to lead with your head when in a hurry, but realize that it's a mental issue that causes your head to go forward. With practice, if you can hold your head back in place, your center of gravity will be stabilized and you'll be able to stretch out your back leg as you step.

If you're balanced you can take large steps, and actually walk faster. This same principle applies to jogging, too.

When wearing high heels, the heel part is not very stable, so one tends to place most of the weight on the balls of the toes. If you put too much weight on the heel you can easily lose your balance, so please be careful.

CHAPTER 4
My Style

For people who think they don't have anything

Are you prepared for life?

When I look back over the last 10 years of my life, the two most important facts are that I have made my own decisions, and that I have learned from my own mistakes.

If I had been completely satisfied with the teachings of my first teacher and hadn't tried to improve, I wouldn't be who I am now.

No matter how wonderful a person may be every human being has flaws. In addition, everyone is different, so once we have learned the basics well, we need to discover what works best for us.

This is how we can best use others' teachings and advice.

Of course, we have to learn the basics properly first. Doing things your own way without first learning the basics could lead to trouble.

Among my students, there are more than a few who think, "I'll be happy if I can just meet Kimiko," "Kimiko will fix all my worries," "Kimiko will save me somehow."

Dependence is of no use. It's not healthy or helpful for either person in such a relationship. Think for yourself, and learn via trial and error. This is important.

I started a Posture Stylist training course in 2006.

It's a half-year course that includes ten days at a training camp for hands-on learning. I developed the course to train new teachers who could teach their own courses based on the posture walking method I developed.

Early on, I made the mistake of sending posture stylists out into the world after only a few days of instruction. It was a mistake I made because I was only half-heartedly committed to the idea of training others in my teaching methods. I feel nothing but regret over those stylists that I sent out into the world unprepared.

The training course I run now is based on what I learned from that mistake. It was a valuable lesson that led to me a curriculum rich in both quality and quantity. The purpose of the course is to raise stylists who deeply understand the influence of posture walking on both our bodies and minds. These stylists are like my daughters.

When I see those daughters worrying or wavering, I feel compelled to give them a helping hand. However, I try not to.

People grow through struggling and by learning from their own mistakes. Everyone has the power to triumph over their trials. So I try to avoid helping those future teachers more than absolutely necessary. This allows them to develop their own power. People find themselves by puzzling through challenges.

When I decided to make walking my life's work, I didn't ask anyone for advice. I only asked my body. Now that I cherish my body, I've found that I can listen to my heart more closely.

If I had talked with someone, and they had said, "You'd better not do that." "It's impossible." "What's the point of starting something like that now?" it would have squashed my resolve. I would probably have agreed, "You're right. I'm so stupid. What was I thinking?"

It's okay to cry. But after that...

When we're worried about something and ask someone for advice, in many cases we're not really seriously worrying. We simply want someone to agree with our own idea.

You make it seem as though you're asking for advice, but

in reality you just want to vent about something. When you have someone who listens to you kindly, one complaint leads to another and it can go on and on.

If you start something because someone else told you to do it, you leave yourself an easy way out if anything goes wrong—you can always blame the person who told you to do it. That means you end up blaming other people for everything bad in your own life.

So try skipping when you are worried about something. I'm not joking.

You can't skip with a scowl on your face, can you?

Since your body and mind are connected, when you want to influence your mind, try moving your body. You are the only person in the world who is authorized to control your body.

If you can't help worrying about something or feeling down, or if you are filled with resentment, please try skipping, with your upper-body held up straight.

Don't you feel like it's ridiculous to keep worrying once you start skipping?

If you shift your body's posture, the posture of your mind will naturally follow suit.

When you want to take action, it's your posture that is important above all else.

If you lift up your body and walk, your mind will cheer up naturally. Because we're human beings, of course we go through times when we want to cry. It's okay to cry. However, after getting it all out in a good cry, puff up your chest and move on.

Balancing home life and a career

At home, I am a mother of two children. No matter how busy I am with work, nobody can change my relationship with my children, and I'd never give that up for anything. Whatever happens, they'll always be my children. I cherish my position as a parent more than anything.

However, being a working mom, it's impossible to do all the housework as well. Whatever I can do, I do 100 percent, but I cut corners when it comes to the things that I can't do perfectly. It's important to develop a sense of how to deal with these things.

You shouldn't feel guilty about not doing what isn't possible for you to do. If you feel guilty about whatever you're doing, your child will learn to feel that it's a negative thing. Therefore, it's important to do what you can with a positive attitude.

"Mom isn't perfect, but she's trying her best for me." Whether your child can think this way or not depends on your attitude, doesn't it?

Your child will understand. They might even come right out and say, "Thanks mom, but don't push yourself."

There are many modern, working women who subscribe to the "should" theory: "I should do this. I should be like this." But we're human beings, not machines. We can't put that much pressure on ourselves.

No one is perfect. When it comes to child care and running a household, it's all right if we do our best within the limits of our power. We don't need to mold ourselves to arbitrary standards set by others' expectations for mothers.

My eldest son entered a high school this year and he asked me if he could dye his hair during the spring holiday. I didn't forbid him from doing it. If I had said "No," someday soon he would have dyed his hair in secret. He wanted to feel satisfied through the action of dying his hair, not necessarily by the end result of his new 'do.

After he dyed it, I gave him my honest opinion. "You know, that color doesn't suit you. Isn't it odd to have black eyebrows with brown hair? Why don't you dye your eyebrows as well?"

After this, he thought about it himself, eventually dyeing his hair back to black. I hope he feels satisfied because he made the decision by himself. It's important for parents to lead their children to think for themselves.

People I work with often ask me, "How do you manage to juggle your career and your household affairs?"

The trick is to admit what you can and can't do, and work within your limits. I remember telling my children, "I'll do the best that I possibly can, so please be understanding. And please do the things that you can do by yourself, on your own."

Trusting your body

I think this story will come as a surprise to anyone who hasn't known me from long ago. I must come clean and tell you that I was in the Japanese Maritime Self-Defense Force (the equivalent of the Navy) for three years after I graduated from high school.

My brother, who is two years older than me, was already serving with the SDF. I thought I'd find a simple job after I graduated from high school.

When my brother was about to take a college entrance exam, my father suddenly developed a duodenal ulcer. He needed major surgery to remove his duodenum and two-thirds of his stomach.

Due to this, my brother had no choice but to give up college and get a job.

Because I had witnessed my brother making such a decision, I felt it would be unfair if I were the only one in the family to go to college.

I spent a tough three months going through physical training at Yokosuka base immediately after I enlisted. The 18- to 19-year-old girls who wanted to join the SDF had come to the base from all over the country. We swam 2 1/2 miles. We rowed boats as fast as we could until our backs were bruised. We painted our cheeks with black ink and crawled on our hands and knees.

We ran 1.3 miles every morning and 2.2 miles every evening.

"What's the point of doing this much exercise, from dawn to dusk?" I complained to an instructor, my bitterness apparent in my voice.

"We all have ups and downs in our lives. This training might seem meaningless at the moment, but the fact that after three months you'll have completed a period of hard training will give you confidence. It will help you deal with anything that comes along in your lives. Do your best, 'cause it's worth it!"

I'll never forget that instructor's words.

It's interesting that while I was running each day I'd think, "I can't go on any more!" But the next morning I was up and at it again.

As the instructor said, I could do it if I tried, and if I tried hard, I'd finish having done my best.

I had the revelation that humans don't die easily, even when they're forced to do very difficult things.

In fact, it was probably the first time that I learned to trust my body and discovered the joy of physical exercise. That whole time is now a pleasant page in my youth that I can flick back to.

After three months at Yokosuka base, I was assigned to a Maritime SDF base in Chiba Prefecture for three years. There was a limit on how much you were allowed to go out if you were stationed at the base. I could not even contact my parents freely because it was in the days before cell phones were prevalent. Because we lived under many restrictions, some of the slightest things provided tons of joy.

For example, we women were cherished like flowers! There were thirty of us working amongst 3000 men. In those days, I didn't dislike strengthening my body in such a Spartan community as the Self-Defense Force. However, if you want a beautiful body, a Spartan regimen isn't the best way to get there.

It's best to have a great time training your body slowly and carefully.

Things given to me by my parents

My father and mother still regularly take a bath together. They say, "We do it because we're worried about the other falling in the tub." They've taken a bath together since I was a child. They are on such good terms it seems as though they can't spend even a second apart from each other.

I've been through a divorce, but I whole-heartedly think that couples supporting each other for a long time are beautiful to behold.

The main gift that my parents gave me that I appreciate the most is my body.

My father was born in the Taisho era, before 1926. He was 5'10" tall when he was young, and because of his build, he was often mistaken as Rikidozan, a famous pro-wrestler. My brother is 5'11" and I am 5'9". This makes me think that I take after my father's side.

My mother is 5'3" and was born in Kyoto. She was a fashion model when she was young. My mother's younger sister—my aunt—was also a model. Everyone in my mother's family was model material, and ever since I was very little I thought that both sisters were very pretty.

When Parents' Day came around at my elementary school, I was so proud that my mother was beautiful. My mother became a housewife after she married my father. I grew up in an ordinary, average home with my family.

Looking back, I probably grew up in a slightly old-fashioned family. My mother always devoted herself to my father from the bottom of her heart. When my mother heard my father returning from work, all of us greeted him at the door. I would untie his right shoelace and my brother would untie the left. While we did so, we sang out "Welcome home!" in concert.

You can't imagine taking part in such a scene yourself, can you? However, I thought it was the norm until very recently. It had been that way since I was little.

There is still an old-fashioned sense in me that a woman should devote herself to her man, and I'm sure that this is a result of my parents' influence. My father wore the pants in the family, and my mother was always careful to show my father in a favorable light. Still, my father always let us kids lead bohemian lifestyles if we wished, never establishing firm limits for us.

As a result I was a tomboy, cheerful and unrestrained during my childhood. My father and mother trusted me in whatever I said or did, and always praised me while I was growing up.

When my father saw an actress on TV, he always said, "Kimiko is prettier than she is." He's a doting father. He says such things to this day.

When I decided that I was going to get a divorce, I called home and said, "There's something I want to talk to you about." I boarded a plane and flew back to my parents' house in Okayama.

When I said, "I'm getting a divorce," my father simply said, "I understand."

"You must have thought it through thoroughly," my mother offered.

Neither of them asked me for any reasons, nor did they try to talk me out of the divorce. Because I had never made any complaints about my married life up until that point, they must have thought that there was a legitimate reason for me to make such a decision.

Then one day, quite some time after my divorce had been finalized, my father and mother asked me, "So why did you decide to get divorced?" It was as if they had only just then thought to ask such a thing.

I think I inherited my present positive mindset from my parents.

How to bring powerful people into your life

When I ponder the meaning of life and its mysterious workings, the first thing that pops into my mind is the idea

with someone who has good fortune, your fortune will improve." But don't you think this disregards the fact that luck is fickle and constantly changing?

Even if you meet a man who appears to be lucky, it's useless to try to take advantage of his luck. The concept of working to enhance your partner's life as well as your own is important. Thinking, "I want to meet my lucky man" or "I want to marry a man with loads of money" is a mistake to start with. If you go into it with such an idea, he may end up deceiving you at some point.

Being with such a partner, relying on his support and riding on his coattails, will eventually become exhausting.

Do you think that if you marry such a person, you'll find happiness? There are very few women who can find happiness pretending to be some celebrity. Love is the pleasure of building up each other's happiness together. If you set a goal and you achieve it easily, will you be satisfied? Do you really expect to find happiness with such an approach to life?

Marriage shouldn't be a goal. Marriage is the beginning of another chapter of your life. This is what I have learned from my own experiences, anyway.

Of course, once you're married, usually your life gets easier, both economically and mentally. But there are also many things that you have to shoulder in married life. There is the pleasure of being together, but there is also the pain of molding yourself into compatibility with your partner. There are always two sides to the coin. I can't stress enough how important communicating is. It's also important to increase your level of tolerance and listening skills. Most importantly, you should form a relationship that will help you and your partner grow as people.

Even if you find your one true love and get married, there are few flawlessly happy marriages where nothing bad happens at all. There's a saying that through marriage, people burnish each other.

Don't be duped by ever-changing fads or trends. When you depend on something, you'll soon lose your confidence in regards to everything else.

I think it's a mistake to live such a life.

If you ask 100 people, you'll get 100 different ideas about love. The media turn each new concept into a catchphrase in order to sell products. That's their job. If you don't have your own strong belief system, you can be easily influenced by mass media and pop culture.

Whose romance is it?

These days, there are many articles in books and magazines that tell you how to become popular with men.

I don't approve of that approach.

I'm not a fan of the type of woman who constantly flatters men. Men might find some such women exciting enough to mess around with, but I think that most men won't care to build a close relationship with them. A successful man will generally choose a woman who can hold a competent conversation while encouraging him to better himself just by virtue of her presence. You'll bore them if you're nothing more than a yes-man (or yes-woman). You can't always be impressed by what they say.

Sure, some men are thrilled when they're told that they are wonderful or amazing. However, they'll get tired of being always told such things. They may enjoy it for a while, but it will not last long.

The secret to succeeding in love is to not lose sight of yourself. First and foremost, ask yourself, "Whose romance is it?" If you only adapt yourself to what you think your partner wants and end up losing your sense of self, you'll end up a slave to love.

If you're not happy, it'll make your partner feel bad. You should work on finding the borderline and striking the right balance between your needs and the needs of the relationship.

A woman who raises a man's "stock"

If you're a woman who is determined to live life well and you're able to have empathy for others, people around you will treat you with respect. There are countless examples of women who ooze charm and have appealingly positive attitudes even if they're overweight or not particularly attractive.

It can be the elegance of your posture, or your ability to show consideration for others by simply saying "thank you" or "I'm sorry" properly, or something like refining your table manners: daily gestures and behavior that we don't give much thought to are in fact very important elements. If you appear to be a refined woman, men will think, "I have to take her to nice places." If you communicate with the staff in a proper manner, he'll think, "I can introduce this woman to my mother, no sweat."

If a man dates a proper woman, his stock rises.

It's not a matter of age, nor is it a matter of having a beautiful body. Focus on developing an inner beauty that creates an aura around you.

The attitude of people around you is a mirror that shows your own reflection

There are various interactions between people in the workplace. You might be asked out repeatedly by a particularly persistent coworker, or you might even become a victim of sexual harassment. However I think that rude or obnoxious types would think twice if your back is held straight and you exude an air of confidence. They'll pounce if they sense weakness in you.

The attitude of people around you is a mirror that shows you your own reflection.

A girl who is pretty and has excellent posture has a stable sense about her. She doesn't open herself up to outsiders. Men wouldn't think of trying to touch you if they're saying, "You always have such great posture."

If someone does touch you, you should say firmly, "What the hell do you think you're doing?" You should look the man straight in the eyes and say, "I am not that easy." My body was loved, respected and taken good care of by my parents. I couldn't forgive myself if I fell prey to a man filled with ugly desire.

You have to realize how important you are and firmly be yourself, with confidence.

Some time ago after giving a lecture, a certain man treated me to a meal and then drove me to my hotel. He seemed like he wanted to come up to my room. I acted with resolution and said to him, "Thank you. I'll say good-bye here." This made him behave in a more gentleman-like manner. He resigned the idea of coming up to my room and said, "Thank you, good night."

To have fortitude is necessary if you want to avoid complicating things with mixed signals or hurting the other's feelings.

Flatly deny them with a smile.

If you stand up for yourself—literally, keeping your posture straight—you'll find you can do your best and clearly say what mean to express.

How to deal with anger

It's important to learn how to clearly and succinctly explain your feelings or problems to others.

When you really cannot or do not want to do something, say so without hiding how you feel about the situation. Express yourself resolutely. It's the best way to be affirmative.

People tend to worry and think, "I might hurt others," or "I should keep my honest feelings to myself." Such wishy-washy thinking leads them to worry needlessly and they eventually end up depressed, thinking they're not good enough. Most often, expressing your feelings directly and honestly is the best way to avoid hurting others, or the best shortcut to solving a problem.

On those occasions, the important thing is to speak slowly and clearly.

If you speak with a low voice, it will sound as though your voice is coming from deep inside your body. You will seem reliable to the listener, whose opinion of you will rise. When you speak slowly and distinctly, you'll find a high-pitched voice doesn't fit.

If you find yourself in a situation where you have to talk in front of a large audience, try to find one person in the audience who seems receptive, maybe who nods as you talk, then direct your speech to that person.

Communicating with just that person is a great way to key into the audience. That one person acts like a proxy for everyone else. This method is a shortcut to communicating with many people.

No matter how much knowledge you have or how good your manners are, though, it's very important to be earnest.

People respond to emotions because we are all emotional creatures. It's doesn't matter whether you're a scintillating conversationalist or not, what matters is that you speak from your heart.

What you intend to express will come across if you say it with feeling. However, if you're full of bitter complaints, you're probably better off not putting those feelings into words.

If you get the words out, your anger will blaze out and it'll only increase your anger. At such times, I try to skip merrily!

Move your body in a way that expresses the opposite of how you are feeling.

Listen to relaxing music, have a nice cup of coffee or treat yourself to dinner at an expensive restaurant. It's a good exercise to shift your anger into a more positive feeling.

The aesthetics of knowing your place

When I hold seminars for the human resources division or do inductee training in a company, for some reason there are always some male employees who're not exactly happy to be doing my workshop. From the beginning to the very end, their expressions clearly show that they're thinking: "What a pain."

At such times, I feel like shouting, "Get out!"

I want to physically throw them out of the workshop.

I think it's great that companies pay to have their employees learn life and business skills, like how to present a business card, how to walk or correct your posture. It's a once-in-a-life opportunity to attain the necessary know-how that is needed to function as a proper member of society.

I'm not saying you should run yourself into the ground for the sake of your company or other such drivel. But there are many people who don't seem to understand or appreciate their situation as an employee. They're paid a salary, while their company offers them the opportunity to study and better themselves.

Unwillingness to participate is contagious. If one person is unwilling, suddenly the ten people closest to him are unwilling as well.

In contrast, someone who is willing to participate and makes requests like, "Kimiko, can you please teach us how to turn next?" makes the whole session more enjoyable for everyone.

At any given seminar or lecture, whether there are just dozens or several hundred people, there are many kinds of individuals present. Some are happy to be there and some are not.

However, I'd want people to give at least some thought as to why they're there.

There aren't many people who can make money purely out of their own talents.

The employees support the company, and the company supports the employees in return.

When you want to appear appealing to others, capitalize on your uniqueness and charm, but in the office, the main emphasis should be on your work.

Given the state the world is in right now, knowing your place is a valuable asset.

The ability to find yourself

Since I promised myself that I would live up to my potential, good things have started to happen one after another. Not only has my body changed, but the trajectory of my life has changed as well.

By not seeking something outside of myself, I noticed that there were countless diamonds sleeping inside of me. I now think that I could die happy because I was able to achieve the biggest purpose of life: finding oneself.

Up until that point, I kept thinking round and round in circles. Then, as I made up my mind and realized my true calling, everything started to go well. Even so, I think the process—the journey—itself is more important than whether you succeed or not.

How did I get here?

The results accumulated naturally while I was going through the process. I think that a person who values the journey will achieve a type of victory, even if the results turn out to be negligible.

Even though getting laid off is obviously not a good result, the experiences you gain from it can be carried with you and will aid you when you get another job.

Try not to be disheartened by some small failure. It's like tripping on a pebble—no need to lose your mind over the little bumps in life. From the moment we are born into this world, everyone is given life equally. The true test is whether you have the capacity to find yourself.

Superheroes have good posture

The people who come to my lessons are mainly female office workers in their 20s or 30s, or housewives that know of my experience struggling to lose weight after giving birth and who want to know how I managed to drop the pounds.

Among them there are students who clearly have psychological issues such as depression.

When I see such a student, I always think to myself, "She must have come here to change something." With this in mind, I work with that person as much as possible, hoping that my lessons will help her. I deliver lessons to such people with something like a prayer in my heart.

When I lead workshops at companies' business training sessions, I'm always secretly pleased to see the middle-aged men getting into it and loosening up. At first everyone seems very embarrassed by the walking exercises. But when I tell them, "You'll be popular with the ladies if you walk like that," they can't help but smile.

Of course, some men seem embarrassed right up to the end. But if they find even a sliver of satisfaction, then I am happy. That's my goal. If the workshop was enough encouragement to get them to start walking in a manner that suits them, then it wasn't for nothing. I never force anyone to do anything, or harshly criticize their efforts.

Everybody comes to the lessons seeking something.

"I hope this lesson will start them on the road toward happiness." I'm always sending out such thoughts to my students.

I train people in Posture Walking and have them teach their own classes. Someday I hope to put a section on Posture Walking in school textbooks.

Teaching proper walking should be part of the school curriculum. It's hard to misbehave when you have good posture, don't you think?

That's why superheroes all have good posture!

When you have good posture, the "heart of justice" in you is activated, and you live with a sense of what is right and wrong. If everyone had that kind of awareness, it might decrease the crime rate!

I want to increase the number of people in the world whose posture—and hearts—are beautiful.

The importance of high-quality sleep

I take numerous business trips. In my bag I carry many things that help me sleep during the journey. This includes things like earplugs, which I use while on a plane or a high-speed train. I carry aromatherapy vials that I can rub onto my skin that act on my lymph nodes. There's herbal medicine in it, and if I put a drop behind each ear, I sleep very soundly.

Fragrances act on the primary olfactory cortex and emotional centers in the brain. I improve my circulation by using a lavender-infused heat pack when I'm in the office. When I place it across my shoulders, its weight is comforting. I warm it up in the microwave, and use it again and again. As it cools it's very refreshing.

I have various other sleep aids I use. Before going to bed, I always turn on a small electric pot with aromatherapy fragrance in it, and turn on some healing music. I'm asleep in seconds.

Since I can sleep soundly on an airplane when I go abroad on business, I don't suffer from jet lag. I'm busy having a good time so I don't care to have jet lag.

In the plane, if I'm awake, I never get bored either. I look forward to watching the in-flight movies. Before a flight to France, I'm thrilled, thinking, "I can watch three movies on the way!" Because I can enjoy myself during the flight, I feel that I profit from the time spent traveling.

My method of dissolving stress

Despite my age, I am often complimented on my skin. I don't do anything special in my skincare routine. It's probably good that I use products that I like, regardless of name, price or brand.

When people talk face to face, their faces move. Taking with people makes your facial expressions more full and vibrant.

I don't have much stress in my professional life, so I don't need to think about ways of relieving stress. I almost never go out drinking. I figure if I have the time for a drink I'd be better off using that time to study anatomy.

I enjoy studying. I also go to museums and window shop. I spend my spare time around beautiful things. The idea of certain places as healing spots seems to be in fashion; I must say that my favorite one is simple: a bathtub. My bed is also more comfortable to me than anywhere else.

When people complain, it's often the case that they just have too much time on their hands.

When you are caught up in something, other things don't seem that important.

When you have a children, a lot of things happen. They

could really hurt themselves. When I'm with my kids, I realize how happy it makes me that they're simply there and alive. I promise myself, "I'll appreciate this boy as long as he lives."

We complain about things only when we're idle.

The drum of the body

No matter how convenient modern life is or how wealth can buy the best of anything, I don't think levels of human happiness and misfortune have changed very much.

Though people live longer than before, many of them live with debilitating disease. There are also people who are physically healthy, but whose souls are dead. They're the ones who complain, "My life sucks."

It all depends on how much you're able to appreciate your life. I think it plays a major part in determining how happy you are.

No one lives forever.

If you can think to yourself, "I had a good life" or "I had a good time" when you are on your deathbed, you've had a wonderful life, wouldn't you say?

I try to live every day and every second to the fullest. If you do this, the vibrations that emanate from your body change, like the sounds of a beating drum.

The human body is a very sacred thing.

Afterword

If you've gotten to the end of this book and are simply thinking, "Since I read this, it's enough," you won't find the positivity switch. You have to be proactive in your own way.

However, if you rack your brain, seriously ponder life and do something positive, you'll find your answers. Human power is something so huge it can't be activated with a half-hearted approach.

I don't intend to give you the impression that you'll gain loads of confidence, your life will change and you'll create a miracle overnight just by straightening your posture and fixing your manner of walking.

During lessons, I never say fake or misleading things like, "If you do this, you'll never have any worries ever again!" It should be obvious why.

However, I try to light people's "happiness fuse" by

teaching that walking is a source of energy and a source of beauty. I think it is my job to inspire.

After each lesson I want my students to take the ideas home and picture themselves in a bright future, and to listen to what their bodies are trying to tell them.

By doing this, you, too, can reawaken the original beauty of your body. Feelings of happiness and contentment will bubble up, affecting everyone around you in a positive way.

I've become convinced of this phenomenon through my own experience.

From children to the elderly, anyone can do it, anytime, anywhere! This is the strength of Posture Walking.

I plan to train many posture stylists who'll be able to spread the circle of lessons throughout the world.

That's my dream.

If we straighten our posture, our society brightens. The flow of positive energy we add to the world is more precious than anything we can buy with money.

I want to play a part in creating such a world.